Did you know ...

People are moving out West to get CBD, when it is available right now where you live

Cannabidiol (CBD) is legal and available in all 50 states without a prescription

CBD is the oil in Charlotte's Web that helps the children with severe epilepsy

CBD has amazing effects on pain, addiction, anxiety, and many other conditions

CBD is responsible for about 80% of the medical effects of medical marijuana

CBD does not get you 'high', it is very safe, and it is not addicting

Learn more ...

Get Off Opioids! ©

Coming Soon!

A new book by Gregory L. Smith, MD, MPH

To learn more or for specific questions regarding CBD and medical cannabis contact Dr. Gregory Smith directly at: drsmith@cannabis-md.com

Or visit his website: http://www.cannabis-md.com

Dedication:

To all those who have taken the time, energy, and oftentimes leaps of faith, to bring *cannabis sativa* out of it's state of scientific suspended animation and back into our medicine cabinets.

Thank you.

Disclaimer:

The information provided in this book is current and vetted as of August 2017. The research and new data coming out about *cannabis sativa* and cannabidiol (CBD) is certain to change. This book is intended to give the reader a baseline framework, to which, they can add additional information as it comes along in the future.

Table of Contents

The medical cannabis refugee

I want to share one powerful story that was a major motivator for me to write this book. My textbook for medical professionals came out about a year ago. I was invited to a large medical cannabis convention in Boston to speak about using CBD for treatment of a variety of conditions. After the lecture I was invited to do a book signing for two hours. I love book signings, they are an opportunity for me to get close and personal with the people who read my book. One particular young mother came up to me to buy the book. She described the hardship of moving from North Carolina to Colorado, so that she could get medical marijuana for her daughter, who had intractable seizures. She said that she was able to get CBD oil in North Carolina by having it shipped legally to her home. However, her daughter's case of epilepsy only responded a little to the CBD only oil. She was able to get a small quantity of whole plant medical marijuana that was very high in the ingredient THCV. She quickly found out that when she added this, her daughter's seizures almost disappeared-from dozens a week, to one every month or so. She also found that rubbing pure THC oil inside her daughter's mouth right after a seizure helped her recover much more quickly from the severe aftereffects of a seizure. Because whole plant marijuana was a criminal offense in North Carolina, she looked over her options, and after discussing it with her husband, they moved the family to Colorado to be able to get convenient and legal access to CBD, THC, and THCV.

This story is important in several ways. It shows that although CBD can be an excellent medication by itself for many conditions, sometimes it is not enough, and doctors and patients need to have access to all of the wonderful oils in marijuana, not just CBD. Second it gives me an opportunity to educate patients and family members about the many other resources that are out there to provide support, ideas, feedback and advice. In each chapter of the book I provide some websites that I have found particularly useful to patients, family members and caregivers.

So you want to learn about cannabidiol (CBD)

Maybe you have heard about the exciting and often novel medical benefits of medical marijuana. However, you are concerned about getting "high" or "addicted" to the THC that is in whole plant marijuana.

Or maybe you live in a state or country where they don't have legal whole plant marijuana, but you are able to legally get cannabidiol (CBD), and want to find out if it may be beneficial to you.

Perhaps you have a family member or loved one that has one of the dozens of medical conditions such as intractable epilepsy, anxiety, chronic pain, arthritis or Multiple Sclerosis, that can respond to CBD and want to learn more about how CBD works and how to use it.

Or perhaps you have already had an opportunity to see how CBD can work and want to get a deeper understanding of CBD.

Finally, you may have noticed that CBD oils and extracts are available without a prescription at stores and online, and want to know why sometimes a doctor's visit isn't required to get CBD.

Unfortunately, you can't ask over 95% of doctors or pharmacists about CBD, because they have had no formal training on medical marijuana, or CBD.

Written by the author of #1 selling medical marijuana textbook:

I am, Dr. Gregory L. Smith, I am a Harvard-trained physician, residency-trained and board certified in Preventive

Medicine. I have been in primary care practice for over 30 years. About 15 years ago I took a course on how to use marijuana medically for a variety of conditions. It occurred to me that there was no science-based textbook about medical marijuana from which medical students and physicians can learn. If a medical professional wanted to learn about medical marijuana, they had to painstakingly research each subject or condition, and read studies, and clinical anecdotes, many of them decades old. So, I spent two and a half years gathering all of the available research, including basic science research in animals and tissue cultures and clinical trials in humans. I synthesized this body of information and wrote, <u>Medical</u> <u>Cannabis: Basic Science and Clinical Applications</u>. This textbook came out in early 2016 and is a best seller among physicians, medical students, nurses, pharmacists and caregivers.

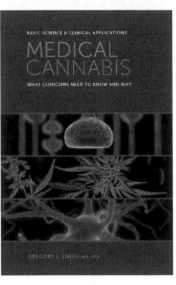

> For more information or to buy the textbook:
> www.aylesburypress.com

Strong resistance from physicians:

Within a few months of publishing my textbook, I realized that the most physicians and medical organizations like the American Medical Association, were still very much against medical marijuana. They felt that there was not enough research to recommend it as a serious medication. There was also still a strong feeling among my fellow physicians that medical marijuana laws were just a means to bypass the prohibition against using marijuana for recreational purposes. This stubborn, resistance to medical marijuana is changing, but very slowly.

In the Spring of 2017, the National Academies of Sciences released the very important, "The Health Effects of Cannabis and Cannabinoids: The Current State of Evidence and Recommendations for Research." This large group of health care providers, and scientists reviewed 10,000s of scientific research and found that medical marijuana was effective in several conditions, and that it may be effective in many more, but research has been significantly hindered by the federal government for the past 40 years.

Profit motivation from pharmaceutical companies

There is very little profit motivation among the larger pharmaceutical companies to spend the millions of dollars necessary to get high quality marijuana-based pharmaceuticals approved by the FDA. The main active ingredients of all marijuana-based medications will be THC and CBD, and they cannot patent these ingredients. Any marijuana-based medication that a pharmaceutical company could patent, could be easily imitated by other companies, without any patent infringement. Without patents, pharmaceutical companies would have a hard time making a profit from these medications.

Smaller more focused pharmaceutical companies, such as G.W. Pharmaceuticals, from the U.K. have approved pharmaceuticals in many countries, and are pending FDA approval in the U.S. of two drugs. It is very interesting to note that the first FDA approval may be for Epidiolex®. This is a $1200-$1800 a month pharmaceutical for intractable childhood epilepsy. It is nothing but 99% CBD extracted from a specific strain of medical marijuana. The very similar 99% CBD extract is available for about $100-$200 a month online or at stores without a prescription. But because it won't be FDA approved it won't be covered by health insurance. But it is still readily available and without a prescription.

How to educate your physician

Physicians are used to being in control of the patient-physician relationship, and to having all of the answers. This creates a significant problem, when 95% of physicians have never taken a class on the Endocannabinoid System (ECS) or have ever learned anything in medical school or residency about using THC and CBD. This is changing, but is will probably be several years before a sizable percentage of physicians and pharmacists have a good working knowledge of medical cannabis or CBD.

The following is website that provides a nice quick summary of the 'pros' and 'cons' of medical cannabis. I have found that if I can get a physician to read this summary, I can quickly get them motivated and excited to learn more.

Have your doctor read this quick and concise article called "The 10-Minute Summary," at ProCon.org.

http://medicalmarijuana.procon.org/view.resource.php?resourceID=142

Empowering People

So while the use of CBD is slowly filtering into the medical community, and small profit motivated pharmaceutical companies are moving ahead with high cost medical marijuana preparations, I felt a strong need to write a concise book that will empower people to take hold of their right to have access to CBD; a legal, effective and very safe medication.

CBD is available without a prescription in all 50 states

After decades with minimal research, there are now over 3,000 studies on CBD, THC and cannabinoids ongoing at this time.

Finally, it is important to learn why and how CBD is legal, and available without a prescription in all 50 states. Even though, most people think they have to visit a physician and be in a state-run marijuana registry to get CBD, this is not true. This book will tell you how, and also how to make certain that you are getting high quality and safe CBD products.

Laws can change, and the current regressive approach on CBD coming out of Washington may lead to limitations on access to CBD. So when you decide to purchase CBD, do some research to make certain that this is legal in your state or country.

Section I: What You Need to Know about CBD

CHAPTER 1

WHAT IS CANNABIDIOL (CBD)

Cannabidiol (CBD) is an oil found in the *cannabis sativa* plant. It is most well known, because it does not have any euphoric effects, it doesn't get you 'high', unlike the other well known ingredient of marijuana, tetrahydrocannabinol (THC.) CBD is especially prevalent in the flowers, or buds. It is also present to a much lesser degree in the stems and stalks of the plant. It is found in high concentrations in certain strains of the plant, and barely present in other strains. CBD is one of approximately 144 cannabinoid oils that can be found only in the cannabis plant. CBD, CBG (cannabigerol) and THC (tetrahydrocannabinol) are the three cannabinoids found in large quantities in marijuana, with many others found in only minute quantities in the plant.

All of the dozens of cannabinoids, other than CBD, CBG and THC are found in only tiny amounts in the plant. Because of this, and due to legal constraints against studying extracts from marijuana, there is very little research or information about the other cannabinoids. Later in this chapter is a list of many of the other lesser cannabinoids, and their potential health benefits. Over the next few years we can expect more research on the health benefits of these other cannabinoids.

This book is predominantly about CBD. However, first I will prove an introduction to marijuana cannabis in general.

Hemp vs. marijuana:

There is considerable confusion, even among people who are intimately involved with marijuana, about the difference between hemp and marijuana. The difference is very important, because in the U.S. when the CBD oil is extracted from research-based hemp plants (less than 0.3% THC) it is considered a nutritional supplement, legal and over-the-counter in all 50 states. However, when the same CBD oil is extracted from non-research *cannabis sativa* plants it is a Schedule I drug, with significant criminal consequences. So the exact same oil can be either an over-the-counter nutritional supplement, or a Class I narcotic, along with heroin, LSD and PCP. There is no medical or scientific reason for this, only politics and financial incentives of powerful pharmaceutical companies.

Both hemp and marijuana, refer to the plant *cannabis sativa.* However, it was arbitrarily decided that if *cannabis sativa* that is less than 0.3% THC by weight, it is hemp and if it is over 0.3% THC then it is marijuana. Hemp has historically been used for millennia for industrial purposes. The plant fiber is used for fabric and rope, and the hemp oil for nutritional and industrial purposes. Whereas, marijuana is used for the oils from the flower or bud, for medical or recreational purposes.

Hemp oil, is the oil that is extracted from non-euphoric hemp plants. This is high in CBD, and very low in THC. CBD oil, is hemp oil that has been further extracted and refined so that there are even higher levels of CBD (3%-99%) and less of the other cannabinoid and terpene oils.

Subtypes of cannabis sativa:

There are two medically important subtypes of *cannabis sativa,* c. *sativa sativa* (sativa,) and c. *sativa indica* (indica). Sativa plants are tall and thin, with long thin leaves, whereas, indica plants are short and stout with short wide leaves. The drawing on the next page is from www.Leafscience.com shows the physical differences of the two subtypes. The ruderalis subtype is not medically important.

Historically sativa and indica grew in more southern parts of the world. The sativa strains typically have high levels of CBD and very low levels of THC. The indica strains have the opposite, much higher levels of THC than CBD. In the past few decades significant cross breeding has led to the development of hundreds of different hybrid strains, which have the characteristics of both subtypes. Strains, colors and aromas do not provide any real information about how potent marijuana is. THC and CBD have no odor. The only real way to know how much CBD or THC is in plant material is to have a laboratory test it.

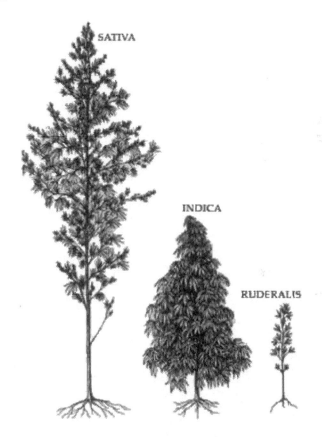

Strains of marijuana:

There are literally hundreds of different strains of marijuana. There are strains that are based solely on the indica subtype, strains based on the sativa subtype, and the newer strains that are hybrids of both subtypes. These strains have comical, and entertaining names, usually based on the fragrance, or color of the crystals in the bud. Some well know examples of strains are Maui Wowie, Blue Dream, Purple Haze, and BC Bud. The variation in aromatic terpenes is a big factor in naming these strains. The terpenes add color and odor to the 'bud.'

The amounts of THC, CBD and terpenes can vary significantly from batch to batch. Just because a strain was mild in one batch, the next batch that is grown can be very different. It is important to look at the laboratory test results from each batch prior to using each new batch of marijuana.

Medical vs. recreational marijuana:

CBD has a much broader impact on health than THC. Some experts believe that 80% of the health benefits from cannabis come from CBD. So marijuana that is to be used for medical purposes should usually be 1:1 ratio of CBD to THC, or higher. There are a few conditions where a higher ratio of THC to CBD is preferred. But generally, when the ratio of THC to CBD gets increased, so do the chances of getting 'high', addicted, or side effects.

The Charlotte's web strain, developed in Colorado by the Stanley Brothers, has a ratio of 20:1, CBD to THC, and less than 0.3% THC. This strain was specifically developed to treat intractable pediatric seizures. There are several other similar strains of high CBD, very low THC marijuana.

Recreational strains of marijuana have much higher amounts of THC than CBD. Since CBD actually diminishes the euphoric effects of getting high, only very small amounts of CBD are usually found in these recreational strains. The most popular recreational strains of marijuana are often 18% or more THC and 0.2% CBD, giving a ratio of 1:90 CBD to THC.

Terpenes:

In addition to the cannabinoids, there are several hundred terpenes that can be found in cannabis. Unlike cannabinoids, which are only found in marijuana, terpenes can be found in a wide variety of plants, herbs, fruits and vegetables. It is often the terpenes that give different strains of marijuana their particular aroma and color. The terpenes are only present in a small amount in the plant oils, but many of the terpenes have their own health effects. However, only beta caryophyllene actually has health effects via one of the same receptors of the endocannabinoid system (ECS) that the cannabinoids use. Beta caryophyllene is found in black pepper, hops, cloves and other plants. It does not cause the euphoria associated with THC, but is more similar to CBD with several medically beneficial effects. Only a handful of terpenes are known to be medically important and are discussed later. All of the important terpenes are available, over-the-counter individually as nutritional supplements.

Flavonoids:

Flavonoids are also present in marijuana oils, as well as all fruits and vegetables. They have potent anti-oxidant effects. In addition, they also contribute to the aroma and color of the plant.

Entourage effect:

Whole plant marijuana oil is made up of a combination of THC, CBD, other cannabinoids, as well as a wide array of terpenes, and flavonoids. Research in the 1980s with pure synthetic THC analogues, without any other cannabinoids or terpenes, has shown that THC works better and in a much more natural way, with far fewer side effects when CBD, and terpenes are present. This synergistic and modifying effect is known as the 'entourage effect'. The presence of CBD, other cannabinoids and terpenes actually makes for a more natural effect on the body's Endocannabinoid System (ECS.)

The entourage effect is used in the development of cannabis-based medications. Often the medications will be shown by the ratio of CBD to THC. For example, the best tinctures for childhood seizures are around between 18:1. That is very high in CBD with only minimal amounts of THC. Pain is usually best treated with 1:1 medication.

THC:

Tetrahydrocannabinol (THC) is the one of the two medically important cannabinoids found in high levels in marijuana. THC is the psychoactive cannabinoid, and is the component in marijuana associated with all of the significant adverse effects. This book is focused on CBD, and I will only briefly discuss THC here. THC is importantly medically, and works differently from CBD, and has a wide array of medical effects that are much different from CBD.

THC is the cannabinoid that is associated with addiction. Using CBD in combination with THC, in 1:1 combination, greatly reduces the THC euphoria, and the chance of developing an addiction.

THC is the cannabinoid that is associated with uncovering psychotic or paranoid behavior. Again, using CBD in combination with the THC greatly reduces the chance of getting psychotic symptoms. In fact pure a dose of 100-200 milligrams of a tincture or vaporizer of CBD can be given to someone having bad effects from recreational marijuana, to rapidly decrease these adverse effects.

Other Cannabinoids:

This book is about CBD, so I will only briefly mention the other cannabinoids. There are about 144 different cannabinoids, so this list just discusses those that are more medically important. The names often sound similar, it is best to use the abbreviation that has been developed for the cannabinoids. All of the cannabinoids interact with receptors of the body's innate endocannabinoid system (ECS) to varying degrees, with varying health and euphoric effects. Again, because of the federal restriction on studying marijuana since 1970, there has been very little research done on these lesser cannabinoid oils.

CBC   -   cannabichromene:

No euphoric effects. May have anti-inflammatory and anti-viral effects, and facilitate pain relief. It also may have anti-depressant effects.

CBG   -   cannabigerol:

No euphoric effects. May promote bone growth, and have anti-inflammatory effects. Being studied for its ability to inhibit tumor and cancer cell growth.

CBN   -   cannabinol:

No euphoric effects. May promote bone growth, and have anti-inflammatory effects. Being studies for helping with sleep.

THCV -tetrahydrocannabivarin:

Intense euphoric effects with lasting shorter duration than THC. Being studied as an appetite suppressant. May promote bone cell growth. May help with tremors and other symptoms associated with Alzheimer's disease. May work synergistically with CBD to reduce seizures/epilepsy.

11-OH-THC -eleven hydroxytetrahydrocannabinol:

Intense euphoric effects. This is not present in the plant, but when the liver metabolizes THC, it turns much of the THC into 11-OH-THC. It is considered the main active metabolite of THC after being consumed in an edible. It is more potent than

THC and crosses into the brain easier than THC. It is associated with increased appetite.

For complete up-to-date patient oriented information on the cannabinoids, and terpenes go to www.Leafly.com/news/cannabis-101

Acidic forms of cannabinoids -

All of the cannabinoids have an acidic carboxylated form, notated by the small letter 'a' after the abbreviation. For example, THCa, CBDa and THCVa. The acidic forms are how the cannabinoids are present in the raw plant material. After decarboxylation via heat or drying of the plant material, the acidic form is turned into the oxidized form. The acidic form usually acts entirely differently in the body from the oxidized form. For example, THCa, does not cause euphoria, and preliminary research suggests that it has many medical uses different from THC. The only way to get THCa or other acidic cannabinoids is to juice freshly harvested marijuana flowers, and drink the fresh juice. If the juice is left for several days it will naturally oxidize from THCa to THC, etc.

Terpenes-

Terpenes are secreted in the same glands in the marijuana flower as the cannabinoids. There are over two hundred terpenes. These aromatic, often pungent oils, are also found in plants, and herbs other than marijuana. They all do not cause euphoria. There has not been much research yet on terpenes, but there is growing evidence of medical benefits from several of the more common terpenes. Terpenes give different strains of marijuana characteristic fragrances and colors. As was mentioned earlier, terpenes interact synergistically with cannabinoids, as part of the entourage effect, discussed above. Here are some of the more common or important terpenes.

Caryophyllene-

Smells like pepper or cloves. Also found in black pepper, cloves and cotton. Unlike any other terpene, it binds to CB2 cannabinoid receptors in the body.

Limonene-

Smells like citrus. Also found in fruit rinds, peppermint and juniper. Has antifungal and antibacterial effects.

Myrcene-

Smells like earthy cloves. Also found in mango, hops and lemongrass. Has sedating, muscle relaxing effects. Myrcene probably responsible for "in the couch" sensation.

Pinene-

Smells like pine needles. Also found in pine, rosemary, basil, and parsley. Counteracts some adverse effects of THC.

How is CBD Extracted:

The oils in cannabis, including the cannabinoids, and terpenes, have been extracted via various methods for over a hundred years. The extracted oils are then further processed to increase the percentage of all or specific cannabinoids. A wide variety of solvents are used to dissolve the oils in the plant material. The type of extraction methodology will determine what contaminants are in the extract. Repeated extraction techniques result in less and less residual plant material, and consequently a lighter and clearer fluid.

Different extraction techniques can absorb different oils from the plant more or less effectively. Olive oil, and ethanol usually extract more of the terpenes than the other solvents.

Hydrocarbon Solvents-

Various hydrocarbons, including benzene, butane, hexane, and propane, can be used to dissolve the oil into a liquid. A slight remnant of these solvents usually remains in the extract. Since these hydrocarbons can contain carcinogens, especially after heating, extracts made using these solvents are not recommended.

Ingestible Solvents-

Several ingestible solvents, such as ethanol, olive oil, coconut oil and butter, can be used to dissolve the cannabinoids into an edible liquid. These are safe and of course edible. However, the food grade oils, are perishable. These extracts are generally made for ingestion as an extract, or in cannabis butter for making edibles.

Carbon Dioxide-

Either supercritical or subcritical carbon dioxide (CO_2) extraction, is currently the safest and most popular means of obtaining high purity extracts. Carbon dioxide extracts an oil which very high in purity and is free from chlorophyll, and most other plant contaminants.

 It is used under high pressure and at extremely low temperatures to isolate the medicinal oils from the contaminants often present with other extraction methodologies. CO_2 extractions are used for an extract that is to be inhaled or ingested.

CHAPTER 2

HISTORY AND LEGAL ISSUES OF CDB USE

This chapter is based on a similar chapter in Dr. Smith's textbook for medical professionals, Medical Cannabis: Basic Science & Clinical Applications from www.AylesburyPress.com. Several paragraphs are used directly from this textbook.

During human evolution many plants have been discovered to have euphoric or medicinal effects. The earliest medications that our ancestors used were from plants, opium for pain, foxglove and digitalis, willow bark and aspirin, cinchonine and quinine. Marijuana with it's often poignant aroma, and rapid onset of effects was bound to be discovered by our ancient ancestors.

Cannabis sativa grows naturally in many tropical parts of the world. Marijuana has been used for its fiber and oil bearing seeds for 11,000 years. Marijuana plants were made into fiber for cloth and rope. The oil from the seeds was used for a variety of household uses.

Ancient use of marijuana:

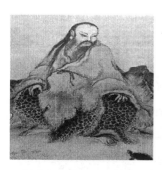

Chinese Emperor FU HSI (2900 BC) recommended medical cannabis

The first recorded medical use of marijuana was described in Indo Chinese medical texts more than 5,000 years ago. At that time it was found to be useful for a variety of both physical and mental conditions. A Chinese medical text of the time prescribed marijuana leaves for tapeworm. The seeds were pulverized and added to wine to help with constipation and hair loss.

Marijuana use for recreational and medicinal effects spread throughout the Greek and Roman empires, and subsequently throughout the Islamic empire. Herodotus in 440 B.C.E., discussed the Scythians using cannabis to make a vapor for steam baths. By the Middle Ages it was regularly used externally as a balm for muscle and joint pain.

Marijuana was introduced to the America's by the Spaniards in 1545 for use as fiber. Hemp became the first major fiber producing plant in the U.S. By 1619 King James I ordered every colonist to grow 100 plants specifically for export. Hemp was a major crop throughout the Americas by the 18th century.

Western medical use of marijuana:

Although, cannabis plants were ubiquitous throughout the U.S., marijuana as a medicine did not make it's way into Western medicine until the 1839. At that time, Dr. William B. O'Shaughnessy returned from India with considerable experience using marijuana for medical purposes. He encouraged physicians to recommend it for insomnia, pain, muscle spasms and other physical conditions. It soon became an accepted treatment.

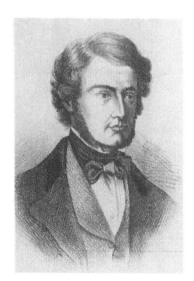

William Brooke O'Shaughnessy

1809-1889

After its introduction and widespread acceptance into medical practice of the time, it started to be used for a wide variety of ailments, including gonorrhea, cholera, whooping cough and asthma. It was predominantly used as an orally ingested tincture. It is said that Queen Victoria used cannabis tincture for menstrual cramps.

Cannabis Indica Tincture

The potency, efficacy and side effects of various medicinal preparations of marijuana extracts varied significantly. For decades these tinctures were sold a "patent medicines" and therefore the ingredients were secret. By the late 19th century laws were already being enacted to address issues with mislabeling, adulteration, and sale of "poisons." In addition, smoking marijuana for recreational use in upscale hashish parlors flourished next to the thriving opium dens of the late 19th century.

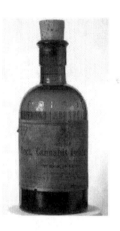

By the beginning of the 20th century laws in several states required prescriptions for marijuana extracts. By this time cannabis was the second most common ingredient in medications and there were over 2000 cannabis containing preparations from over 280 manufacturers.

U.S. Marijuana laws:

The Pure Food and Drug Act of 1906, and several state's laws were passed to restrict "habit-forming drugs." These were the start are a series of laws to control, and regulate drugs.

In addition smoking cannabis for the first time was becoming popular in the population because of over a decade of alcohol prohibition. This lead to a backlash against smoking cannabis, which was previously acceptable only among Mexican migrant workers and Negro Jazz musicians. The term "marihuana" later changed to marijuana, was a slang term used by Mexican immigrants to describe cannabis, it meant "Mary Jane" in Spanish. The federal government began use the term marijuana in all government documents, to separate 'smoked' marijuana from the very popular *cannabis sativa* elixirs that were used medicinally. The movie "Reefer Madness" (1938) is a classic example of this hysteria of this era.

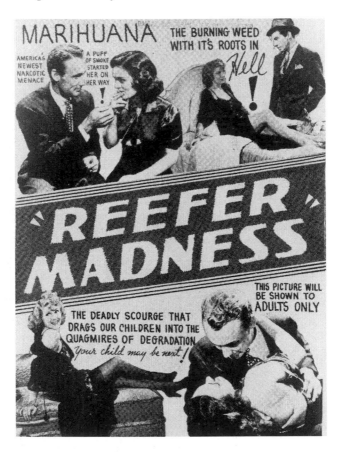

At the same time, the Marijuana Tax Act of 1937 imposed a levy of one dollar per ounce on marijuana used for medical use and $100 per ounce for recreational use. This law effectively made non-medical or non-industrial use, possession or sale of marijuana illegal throughout the U.S.. At that time the fledgling American Medical Association (A.M.A.) was against this law, and correctly thought that it would impede future research into the drug. By 1938 the Federal Pure Food, Drug and Cosmetics Act established the framework that we still use today to regulate prescription and non-prescriptions drugs. By 1951 the Boggs Act, added *cannabis sativa* to the list of narcotic drugs.

The use of marijuana for medical purposes dramatically decreased over the course of the early twentieth century. There was some research in the 50's and 60's for use in glaucoma. But far superior ophthalmic medications became available.

THC was not isolated from *cannabis sativa* until Dr, Raphael Mechoulam discovered it in Israel in 1964. CBD had been isolated several years earlier, along with dozens of other cannabinoids. In the 70's a synthetic version of THC called Marinol(R) was approved for chemotherapy induced nausea and vomiting and later for cancer and AIDS-related wasting syndrome. The intense euphoric side effects from pure THC and need to swallow oral capsules while nauseous made this a poor clinical choice. The advent of superior medications has made almost use of synthetic THC pharmaceuticals obsolete.

In 1969, during a very turbulent period of "anti-war" social unrest, president Nixon pushed for a comprehensive restructuring of drug laws, for what he called, "a war on drugs." He was especially focused on marijuana because of its association with the "anti-war" movement. The Controlled Substances Act (C.S.A.) was passed as part of the Comprehensive Drug Abuse Prevention and Control Act of 1970, This made the possession or distribution of *cannabis sativa* criminal at a federal level. This legislation created the five Schedules of Dangerous Drugs. The Drug Enforcement Administration (D.E.A.) and Food and Drug Administration (F.D.A.) together were to determine which drugs are placed into the Schedules. It placed cannabis into Schedule I, where the drug was determined to have no medical use and had a high risk of addiction.

See the following website for the current status of marijuana and CBD laws in the US.
www.wikipedia.org/wiki/Legality_of_cannabis_by_U.S._juri sdiction

CBD research:

This legislation effectively put an end to all serious scientific study of medical marijuana, including CBD and severely limited the study of the cannabinoids. In the early 1990's the Endocannabinoid system (ECS) was discovered. We learned that cannabinoids have their effects in the body by binding to natural cannabinoid receptors in the brain and body that make up the ECS. Since this natural system in our body was discovered, researchers have conducted tens of thousands of studies in animal models and tissue culture on the effects of the various cannabinoids. However, the main research on CBD in humans has been done by GW Pharmaceuticals in trials for children with rare intractable epilepsy. CBD is one of the three cannabinoids present in high quantities in marijuana, and a growing body of research has shown how CBD can have a wide array of beneficial medical effects.

U.S. medical marijuana laws:

After several failed attempts, California was the first state to pass Proposition 215 in 1996, known as the Compassionate Care Act. This along with Senate Bill 420 in 2003 allowed for a network of growers, caregivers, healthcare providers and an identification card system for medical marijuana. As of the time of this writing 42 states and the District of Columbia have some sort of legalized medical cannabis laws.

Whole plant versus CBD only laws:

Whole plant marijuana refers to having measurable quantities of THC, so that there may be euphoric effects. Many of the states allow for CBD only, which means the plant or extract has very low amounts of THC, and high amounts of CBD. Charlotte's web is an example of a strain of marijuana that is very low in THC and high in CBD. Most of the laws that allow for CBD only, state that this medicine can be used to treat intractable seizures only.

Some countries have taken a much more practical approach to defining medical marijuana. In these countries as long as the ratio of CBD to THC is 1:1 or greater (higher in CBD) then it is considered legal for medical use. This is a wise approach as CBD significantly decreases the euphoric effects of THC, and CBD blocks almost all of the adverse side effects, like paranoia, anxiety, agitation and addiction, that come from THC. Very importantly, it is unusual from a patient to become addicted or dependent from the use of high CBD marijuana.

The regulations and requirements vary considerably among the states and countries. For example, New York allows for medical marijuana, as long as it isn't smoked. Some allow only for the use of medical marijuana for Qualified Conditions (QC) such as Multiple Sclerosis, or Alzheimer's disease. The QC vary considerably from state to state, and are based on political and not scientific motives. That being said, the generally recognized efficacy of THC and CBD and the innate safety of these drugs has underpinned the support and continued expansion of medical marijuana laws in the U.S. and around the world.

Changes in federal marijuana policy:

In 2009 based on the rapidly evolving changes at the state level in legalization of medical cannabis, the U.S. Attorney General stated, "It will not be a priority to use federal resources to prosecute patients with serious illnesses or their caregivers who are complying with state laws on medical marijuana, but we will not tolerate drug traffickers who hide behind claims of compliance with state law to mask activities that are clearly illegal."

In December 2014, congress and the Obama administration quietly put an end to the federal prohibition against medical cannabis as a tiny part of a federal spending bill. However, federal banking laws still force medical dispensaries to operate as "cash only" businesses.

Most recently the prescription opioid epidemic that has been ravaging the U.S., has helped push cannabis into the spotlight as a much safer and less toxic alternative to opioids for pain control. Cannabis has been shown to be very helpful with transitioning patients off opioids.

The F.D.A. Continues to have *cannabis sativa* as a Schedule I drug, but there are major efforts underway to reschedule to a lower schedule drug classification, or perhaps deschedule marijuana as a medicine, and instead treat it like alcohol or tobacco regulated substances.

U.S. CBD laws:

Cannabis sativa, and any extracts from the plant are still an illegal drug at a federal level in the US, and require a doctor's recommendation letter in those 29 states where it is legal. Even extracts of pure CBD, if they originated in the flower of the non-hemp *cannabis sativa* plant, are considered illegal drugs. Only CBD oil that originated in legal hemp plants is legal and available online and in all 50 states.

On February 7, 2014, President Obama signed the Farm Bill of 2013 into law. Section 7606 of the act, Legitimacy of Industrial Hemp Research, defines industrial hemp as distinct from marijuana and authorizes for the first time since 1937 in the US for institutions of higher education or state departments of agriculture in states that legalized hemp cultivation to regulate and conduct research and pilot programs. So far 31 states that defined industrial hemp as distinct from marijuana, and removed barriers to it production. This has led to a plethora of high quality, US grown hemp oil available.

To further support the intent of the 2014 Farm Bill, and stop efforts by the DEA to control CBD and the expanding state medical cannabis laws the Appropriations Act of 2017, Sec 773, explicitly states that federal funds may not be used to:

"prohibit the transportation, processing, sale, or use of industrial hemp that is grown or cultivated in accordance with section 7606 of the Agricultural Act of 2014, within or outside the State in which the industrial hemp is grown or cultivated."

So the legal over-the-counter CBD products are manufactured from legal cultivated hemp, are exactly the same as CBD from other sources.

CBD Laws in other countries:

Pure CBD, or low-THC hemp oil is generally not considered a scheduled substance, or an illegal drug anywhere in the world. It is generally considered to be hemp oil, a cosmetic ingredient or nutritional supplement. However, in some countries, it is considered to be a controlled substance, requiring a prescription from a physician.

Epididolex®:

An UK-based pharmaceutical company has been developing several marijuana-based prescription medications over the past 20 years. One of these meds Epidiolex® it is a 99% CBD, extracted from the flowers of a specific strain of *cannabis sativa*. It has recently been given and "orphan drug designation" by the FDA for the treatment of two very rare forms of childhood intractable seizures. This means that this drug may very soon become available by prescription in the US for these conditions. It will probably cost $18,000-$30,000 a year for this prescription medication, unlike other better whole plant CBD extracts that are readily available online or in stores for around $1200 a year.

The recent FDA recognition of this 99% pure CBD as an Independent New Drug may result in it becoming a prescription medication. This has created great concern among the many of the manufacturers of other high concentration CBD extracts that sell their products. They may have to stop selling or producing their products if this is causing patent infringement or other legal issues with the manufacturers of Epidiolex®. This is a very recent development at this time. Readers can Google Epidiolex® to learn more.

Physician education and cannabinoids:

It is estimated that about one percent of physicians in the US regularly recommend medical marijuana in their practice. About five percent have had any education on the endocannabinoid system (ECS) or training on the use of cannabinoids such as THC and CBD oil. There are several reasons for this. Even though marijuana has a long and respected history as a medicine, it was not until the early 1990's that the ECS was discovered, and researchers could start to evaluate how cannabinoids work in the brain and body. So most of today's practicing physicians were already out of medical school while the ECS was first being discovered and researched. Not unexpectedly there is essentially no consistent training or education of medical students, even to this day, on cannabinoids, medical marijuana or the ECS.

The first medical marijuana law passed in California in 1996, and the perception of the medical community, has been that medical marijuana laws were ways for people to bypass the prohibition against the recreational use of marijuana. Indeed, in many states there is strong evidence to suggest that medical marijuana laws are facilitating recreational users getting easy access to relatively inexpensive marijuana.

Finally, *cannabis sativa* was put into Schedule I of the federal Controlled Substances Act in 1970. This federal law described marijuana as having no medical benefits and being highly addictive. Being in Schedule I severely limited human research on cannabinoids for the past 40 years. Almost, all of the research in humans is either very old, from the 70s and 80s, small poor quality studies, or were done using synthetic pharmaceuticals and not whole plant marijuana. Just in the past few years have high quality, whole plant marijuana studies in humans started to be published.

I wrote my textbook, Medical Cannabis: Basic Science and Clinical Applications (2016) (http://www.aylesburypress.com) because there was no science-based text available to educate medical students, physicians and other medical professionals on medical marijuana.

CHAPTER 3

CBD: How Does CBD Work?

CBD is a very safe and effective with few adverse effects. It has many medical effects in the brain and body, and works on many medical conditions. CBD is probably responsible for 80% of medical effect. Unlike, THC, there is no euphoria associated with CBD, and no concern about addiction or dependency. In general CBD can be considered an adjunct, or helper, to be used in conjunction with other medications that are already available. In the future CBD may be considered a preventive medicine, and taken in a small, once-a-day dose to prevent or slow the progress of a wide array of chronic degenerative conditions.

Endocannabinoid system (ECS):

Like THC and the other cannabinoids, CBD works by impacting the body's Endocannabinoid system (ECS) in several different ways. The ECS is a natural system in our brain and body. It is a system that is present in all animals and fish, and evolutionarily dates back 600 million years. The ECS's job is to modulate other systems in the body that can become overheated. It is like a braking system, that can slow down a wide variety of systems in the body, including pain perception, gastrointestinal motility, memory, sleep, response to stress, pain and appetite, to name a few. The ECS has unique functions throughout the body, but especially in the brain and the immune system. In fact, ECS receptors are the most common receptors in the brain and the second most common receptors in the body, showing exactly how important is the ECS.

Nerve cells, called neurons, release chemical messengers called neurotransmitters. There are literally hundreds of different neurotransmitters released in the body depending on what system is involved. When there are too many chemical messengers being released, and a specific system in getting out of control, the ECS releases, on demand, its own specific chemical messengers to slow down the release of these chemical messengers. So the ECS keeps several of the body's system in balance. The ECS uses two different chemicals, anandamide (ANA) and 2 arachidonoylglycerol (2-AG.) These two chemicals are called endocannabinoids, they are the innate cannabinoids made by the body naturally. These endocannabinoids work by attaching to a cannabinoid receptor on the cell. THC and CBD work by imitating the body's naturally occurring endocannabinoids.

There are two ECS receptors that we know of, that are named simply, cannabinoid receptor 1 (CB1) and cannabinoid receptor 2 (CB2.) There are probably a few more, but these have not been discovered yet. Some systems in our brain and body have CB1 receptors, some have CB2, and some have both.

Much as a lock can only be opened once the key is put in. The lock is the cannabinoid receptor on the cell membrane, and the key, is the endocannabinoid chemical, ANA or 2-AG. Once the endocannabinoid is released, it is quickly broken down by enzymes in the area, so that the effect is only short lived, maybe milliseconds, and only when the endocannabinoids are released.

Endocannabinoid receptors:

Once inhaled or ingested the plant-based cannabinoids present in marijuana, known as phytocannabinoids, get into the bloodstream and travel all over the brain and body. These phytocannabinoidss then bind to CB1 and CB2 receptors in the brain and certain organs in the body just as ANA 2-AG do. This results in similar effects to the body's endocannabinoid chemicals, 2-AG and ANA. When we use medical marijuana we can have much higher doses of cannabinoids, than our body is able to make, thus, getting a medical or therapeutic effect. There are no specific enzymes in the body to immediately break down the cannabinoids from marijuana, so the effects last much longer.

Different cannabinoids in marijuana, interact directly or indirectly with the CB1 and CB2 receptors. The way in which the cannabinoids interact with these receptors, determines what medical effects and what adverse side effects we can expect.

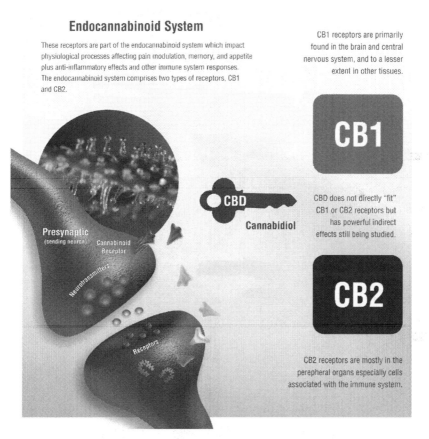

Endocannabinoid System

These receptors are part of the endocannabinoid system which impact physiological processes affecting pain modulation, memory, and appetite plus anti-inflammatory effects and other immune system responses. The endocannabinoid system comprises two types of receptors, CB1 and CB2.

CB1 receptors are primarily found in the brain and central nervous system, and to a lesser extent in other tissues.

Presynaptic
(sending neuron)
Cannabinoid Receptor
Neurotransmitters
Receptors

CBD
Cannabidiol

CB1

CBD does not directly "fit" CB1 or CB2 receptors but has powerful indirect effects still being studied.

CB2

CB2 receptors are mostly in the pereipheral organs especially cells associated with the immune system.

This graphic is from www.canna-pet.com. It shows how CBD works with the ECS.

In general CBD does not directly interact with the CB1 or CB2 receptors, but instead blocks an important enzyme that breaks down our natural cannabinoid ANA. So CBD results in an increase of our naturally occurring cannabinoids, throughout the brain and body. This can be thought of as increasing our cannabinoid tone.

CB1 receptors:

The CB1 receptors are mostly found in certain brain centers. Here is a list of most of the brain centers and their associated function:

Hippocampus - Learning, memory, stress related to adverse memories

Hypothalamus- Appetite

Limbic System- Anxiety

Cerebral Cortex- Pain processing, higher cognitive functions

Nucleus Accumbens- Reward and Addiction

Basal Ganglia- Sleep, movement

Medulla- Nausea and vomiting chemoreceptor

However, there are quite a few organs in the body that also have CB1 receptors including the uterus, cardiovascular system, adipose tissue, gastrointestinal tract, pancreas, bone and liver. We are still learning exactly how the ECS modulates these organs.

CB2 receptors:

The CB2 receptors are found mostly in the immune system cells in the brain and body. These cells are involved with immunity and inflammation. The cells with CB2 receptors include monocytes, macrophages, B-cells, T-cells, and thymus gland cells. These have to do with modulating the release of chemicals involved with inflammation, swelling, immune response, cell migration and programmed cell death. In general when the receptors are activated the immune or inflammatory response is turned down.

CB2 receptors are also found in our bone's osteoblast cells. These cells work in tandem with osteoclasts to create new healthy bone cells. Studies have shown that activation of CB2 receptors results in improved healing of fractures.

Many tissues or organs of the body have both CB1 and CB2 receptors, providing different, often counter-balancing functions. Some of these include: skin, brain, liver, and bone.

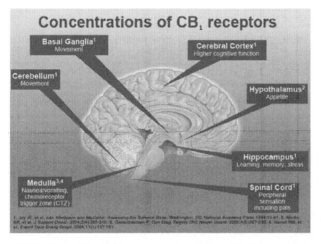

This graphic is from www.theleafonline.com
shows CB1 receptors in the brain.

Change in number of receptors:

The number or density of these ECS receptors, shaped like little buttons, in the membrane of a cell determines by how often the receptors are activated. If over time, there is excess of stimulation of these receptors, then the number of receptors on the cell membrane will tend to decrease, this is called down-regulation. Therefore, it will take more of the cannabinoid to get the same effect. If there is not enough stimulation of these receptors, over time, the number of receptors will tend to increase, this is called up-regulation. This will result in more effects from lower doses of cannabinoids.

In order to learn how to dose CBD effectively, it is important to understand the importance of finding just the right dose that does not result in up- or down-regulation of the receptors on the cell membranes.

THC:

When THC binds to the receptors, it only partially opens the lock. This is called being a partial agonist. THC binds to both CB1 and CB2 receptors. The euphoric effects of THC are due to the CB1 binding in certain brain centers. THC is one of the few well studied cannabinoids that has consistent binding on CB1 receptors.

CBD:

CBD works via the ECS, but unlike THC, it does not directly bind to CB1 or CB2 receptors. Instead it indirectly increases the activity of CB2 receptors. It does this by blocking a certain enzyme known as FAAH. By blocking this enzyme there is an increase in the amount of ANA, one the body's innate endocannabinoids. The net results in increase in CB2 activity. CBD also activates other receptors in the body's systems that have to do with pain perception, and inflammation.

Other effects:

The vast majority of marijuana's medical effects, occur by impacting the ECS. However, the cannabinoids in marijuana have other beneficial therapeutic effects, that don't work through the ECS. Cannabinoids are potent antioxidants and can have effects by counteracting the adverse effects of oxidative stress. In addition, THC has been shown to block the effects of certain enzymes, and have beneficial effects in this way as well. Also, as discussed above, CBD can bind to receptors on cells that are not part of the ECS.

Taking medical marijuana medication:

There are many ways to get cannabinoid medication into the body. The way that the cannabinoid makes it into the bloodstream, and from there to the brain and the rest of the body is very important. There are four main means of taking the medication, inhaling, ingesting, mucous membrane absorption and topically.

Inhalation:

Inhaling implies smoking or vaporizing bud, hashish or oil. When the material is smoked, it is actually combusted, and many products of combustion go along with the vaporized oil into the lungs. Only about 20% of the "smoke" is actually the oil, the remainder is a hodgepodge of potentially carcinogenic hydrocarbons, and inert plant particulates. However, several good studies have failed to find an association with long term smoking of cannabis and increased rates of respiratory tract cancer. It is felt that the anti-cancer effects of THC, and CBD probably cancel out the adverse effects of the carcinogens. However, this matter has not been clearly settled with high quality studies.

When the bud, hashish or oil is heated to a certain temperature (usually around 320-360 degrees Fahrenheit) there is no combustion, there is only vaporization of the cannabinoids and terpenes along with a very small quantity of potentially carcinogenic hydrocarbons present in the plant material.

Smoking cannabis results in incineration of half of the bud, so that only half of oils make into the inhalation into the lungs. Vaporizing is much more effective, as much as 90% of the THC and CBD oils make it into the inhalation into the lungs.

Inhalation leads to direct and rapid entry into the bloodstream via the lungs. It results in effective concentrations of cannabinoids in the bloodstream within a few minutes and maximum effect within 15 minutes. However, beneficial effects only last 60-90 minutes. Because of its rapid entrance into the body, inhalation is good for immediate relief of pain, inflammation or spasm. An inhaled dose usually starts having effects within minutes and usually lasts about one to one and a half hours.

Ingestion:

Ingestion implies eating, drinking or swallowing droplets of a tincture or an extract into the mouth. The medication is usually extracted with coconut or olive made into an extract or with alcohol and made into a tincture. There are also infused drinks, cooked or baked edibles. The medication has to go through the stomach, and into the small intestine where it is metabolized by the liver, before getting into the bloodstream. This process is much slower, with the onset of action taking 1 ½ to 2 hours from ingestion. This slow onset is known as the "first-pass effect" and is a phase that you may hear often. It refers to the fact that when a medication is swallowed it goes into the intestine, and is passed through the liver. In the liver the CBD and THC are metabolized to different chemicals, THC is metabolized to 11-OH-THC, and CBD to 7-OH-CBD and CBD-7-oic acid. The end result for CBD is that only about 15% of it is available after it goes through the liver, the rest has been broken down into inactive metabolites. Also, 90% of the THC and CBD are metabolized into other chemicals via the 'first pass effect". In the case of THC, it is metabolized into 11-OH-THC. 11-OH-THC is actually a much more potent than regular THC.

So the effects of ingested vs. inhaled cannabis medication can be quite different. In addition, ingested cannabinoids work for much longer than inhaled cannabinoids. An ingested dose can last up to 6 hours in the body. Ingested medication is particularly useful for chronic, constant pain or inflammation or for use at bedtime to get relief all night long.

Mucous Membrane absorption:

There are several preparations of cannabinoid medications that are meant to be absorbed via a mucous membrane, the nose, the mouth cavity, or the rectum. For the nose and mouth it is usually in the form of a spray or mist, which is inhaled through the nose or sprayed inside the mouth. For the rectum, it is usually a rectal suppository. When cannabinoid medication is meant to be taken in this way, it is usually absorbed into the bloodstream through local absorption through thin and very vascular mucous membranes. So these medications tend to get absorbed more quickly than ingesting them, and tend to work longer than inhaled medications. They are absorbed within 30 minutes, much faster than edibles, and they last 2-3 hours, shorter than an edible. However, there is no "first-pass" effect, so they are not broken down into metabolites right away, as edibles are.

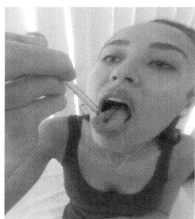 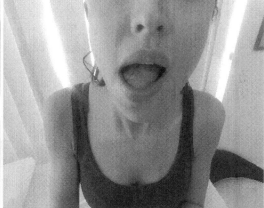

Photograph I   Photograph II

Extracts and tinctures can function as two different medications. Slow release or fast release. If the extract is placed on the tongue (see photograph I) and then swished around the front of the mouth with the tongue (see photograph II), then it will absorb rapidly and miss the 'first-pass effect.' This results in rapid onset of symptom relief, that lasts 1-2 hours. If the same extract is swallowed immediately, or put in a tea and ingested, then it will go through the 'first-pass effect' and both absorb more slowly and last much longer.

Applying to the skin:

Topical application of cannabinoid medications can work in one of two ways. They are either meant to be a salve,

where they are absorbed only locally by painful or inflamed tissues. For example, over a painful arthritic joint or inflamed skin conditions. Often these salves are combined with other active ingredients like camphor, menthol and capsaicin, which also have local effects on pain and inflammation.

There are other topical cannabinoid medications, sometimes gels and sometimes patches, that are meant to result is a constant slow absorption of cannabinoids through the skin and into the bloodstream. These topical cannabinoids have a very slow onset of action, and result in a constant low level of cannabinoids medications for up to 24 hours with one application. However, the absorption is highly variable from person to person.

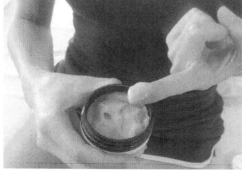
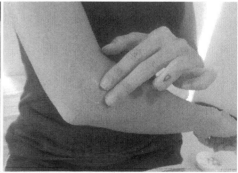

Photograph III   Photograph IV

There are plenty of CB1 and CB2 receptors in the skin, in the tissues immediately under the skin, and around joints of the hands, feet, elbows, knees, and shoulders that can will absorb CBD that is applied topically over a local area. Use a small amount, the size of a dime (see photograph III.) Rub it in with deep pressure, to leave a thin layer over the inflamed skin or joint (see photograph IV).

Forms of the medication:

It is important to have a working knowledge of how the medication can be purchased for use online, or at a store, without a prescription in all 50 states. As was discussed previously, the CBD oil in the legal product must originate from hemp, either hemp from outside of the US, or hemp grown in the US legally under the 2014 Farm Bill. Unless you are in a state with legal medical cannabis, in this case the CBD can come from any source, hemp or marijuana plants.

There are several websites that may be useful to find legal CBD either at a nearby location, or for online purchase. Here are a few

http://www.TheHempDepot.org

www.CBDoilreviews.com

www.CWhemp.com

Flowering Bud

In general *cannabis sativa* bud that is very high in CBD and has less than 0.3% THC, will only be available to purchase in a dispensary in a state that has medical or recreational cannabis laws. It is in general not legal to get high CBD/low THC bud online or in non-legal states. In non-legal states usually extracts, tinctures, various types of edible and vaporizers are available in stores or online.

Even with the dozens of other means of ingesting cannabis, smoking is still by far the most common, even for medical use. I believe that everyone should be familiar with the fat, green 'bud' that is associated with marijuana. Different strains of cannabis have been bred over the decades that have focused on maximizing the percentage of THC and/or CBD in the bud.

There are literally hundreds of different strains of cannabis, with new ones being produced regularly. Some examples of high CBD/low THC strains are, Charlotte's Web, AC/DC, and Cannatonic. Many strains are often named after the aromas given off by the terpenes in the bud, or by the color of the cannabis resin glands called trichomes.

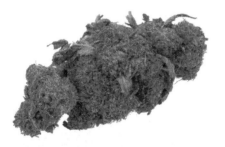

A bud of marijuana

The different strains of cannabis at a dispensary will often have a label stating the concentrations of THC and CBD. The clinician and patient should be aware that these labels are notoriously inaccurate. Each new batch of bud may have markedly different potency, even if it came from the same dispensary and has the same

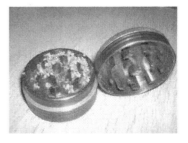

Photograph V

name of strain. Stick the therapeutic goal of starting out with a low dose, and titrate slowly up to clinical effect.

The bud is usually ground in a handheld grinder (see Photograph V) available at dispensaries for a few dollars. Grinding the bud into small particles make it smoke more evenly and smoothly. When the bud is heated up by a vaporizer or burned the crystallized oil releases a fume or vapor of medication that is inhaled. The ground bud can then smoked in rolling paper. The average joint has approximately 400-500mg of dried ground bud in it (see Photograph VI.)

There are a myriad of glass and metal pipes, and water pipes, that are available (see Photograph VII.) These hold large amounts of ground cannabis bud, and are not generally good for use for medication purposes.

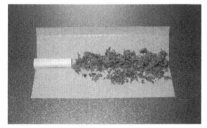

Photograph VI

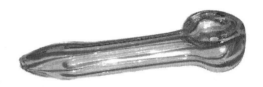

Photograph VII

There are large tabletop or large handheld vaporizers that can cost hundreds of dollars. These allow for strict control of the temperature so that the oils are aromatized at exactly the correct temperature. There are small pen vaporizers, similar to e-cigarettes (see Photograph VIII.) Disposable cartridges are available containing exact amounts of CBD or whole plant extract. Generally, each inhalation of a pen vaporizer will provide 2.0 – 2.5mg of CBD.

These devices vaporize CBD or whole plant (THC and CBD) oil that has been diluted in glycerine or propylene glycol. Propylene glycol is not recommended as a diluent because of health risks associated with it when it is heated.

CBD oil boils at 160-180 degrees Celsius (320-356 Fahrenheit) and turns into a vapor. Whereas THC oil boils at 157

Celsius (315 Fahrenheit). A joint, however, can reach 2000 degrees Fahrenheit incinerating at least half of the bud, before releasing any of the oils for inhalation.

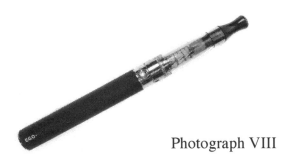

Photograph VIII

Micro-dose Inhaler (MDI):

More recently, the CannaKit® was created with a patented micro-dose inhaler (MDI®). The MDI has the appearance of a cigarette (see Photograph IX) but it is actually a patented metal tube, that tip of which holds exactly 50mg of ground bud. This allows for precise dosing of cannabis medication from 0.5mg to 6.0mg of inhaled medication. It also dramatically reduces the amount of expensive bud that is often wasted with other means of smoking. It comes with an odor-proof carrying case, which carries a couple days of ground bud, and a cleaning tool.

The clinical effects of the medication are directly related to the amount of fume that the patient inhales. The patient holds the inhaled fume in the lungs for 2-3 seconds, to maximize absorption of the medication from the fume in the lungs. The patient is usually advised to start with a small, deep inhalation of the fume. When there is THC in the bud, the initial effects of the medication are usually some euphoria, and these can start within a couple of minutes after this initial dose. Since CBD has no euphoric effects, there are no obvious sensations or effects initially. CBD reaches a peak dose in the blood after about 9-23 minutes, it is at this time that the relaxing, anti-anxiety effects become noticeable. Because the medication is inhaled and bypasses the liver first-pass effect that occurs with eating or swallowing the medications, it starts working much more quickly, but also last a much shorter duration, one to one and a half hours.

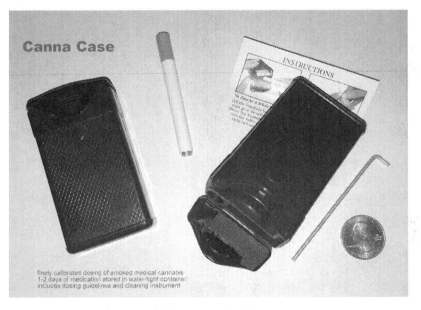

Photograph IX

Learn more at:
www.cannabis-md.com

Smoking or vaporizing cannabis is most useful for episodic need for the medication for acute flare-ups of pain, spasms, seizures, and anxiety.

Smoking bud for medical purposes has several pitfalls. The first is the obvious often intense lingering aroma that is associated with the exhaled smoke. Since cannabis is still usually an illegal drug when used for non-medical purposes this can lead to legal and social issues. The second pitfall is that the cannabis smoke is made up of hundreds of by-products some of which are known respiratory tract irritants, so that the clinician wouldn't want to recommend use of smoked bud in patients with certain respiratory tract conditions, or for use in and around children or people with respiratory tracts conditions.

It is important to note, however, that the smoke-related by-products have not been associated with increased rates of respiratory tract cancer. Also, vaporizing the bud at lower temperatures, instead of igniting the bud when smoking it, releases much higher concentrations of the pure medicine, and markedly less by-products.

Hashish

This is made from the compressed resin glands of the cannabis bud. It contains all of the same active ingredients as the bud, but is more concentrated. The exact hardness of the hashish varies significantly, depending on how it is prepared.

It can be hard and waxy, soft and pasty or come as an oil. The color ranges from earthy browns, to tan and yellowish red (see Photograph X.) It has been around almost as long as humans have been smoking cannabis, and has a long history of medical use.

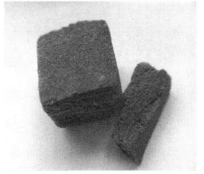

Photograph X

The ground bud can be smoked or vaporized. It is titrated at the same intervals as smoking bud. It is a much more concentrated form of cannabinoids and terpenes, than the bud and the dose needs to be adjusted so as not to get too much medication with each inhalation.

Cannabis bud and hashish are traditionally smoked or vaporized. There are no common CBD only varieties of hashish at this time.

Cannabis Oil

This is a highly concentrated form of cannabinoids in the oil base made by solvent extraction. They usually come in potency from 60-85 percent cannabinoids, but have been reported to be as high as 99 percent cannabinoids (see Photograph XI.) The oil can be consumed as an edible, but traditionally it is vaporized in a specially designed device that produces the very high temperatures necessary for vaporization of the extract for inhalation. This is a much higher temperature than is required to vaporize oil in diluents. Cannabis oils usually contain high amounts of THC and are used for recreational purposes. This formulation is very potent, and complex to administer with huge potential of excessive euphoric effects and side effects from the THC and is therefore, not recommended for medication administration.

The one exception is Rick Simpson Oil. Which is very high in THC and used for 60-90 days to treat late stage cancer. (https://www.leafly.com/news/cannabis-101/what-is-rick-simpson-oil)

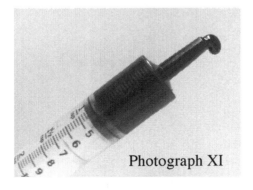

Photograph XI

Cannabis Tinctures and Extracts

Cannabis tinctures are alcohol extractions, the other vehicles for extracting that include coconut and vegetable oils. These liquids contain concentrated CBD or THC and CBD, but also all of the other important organic chemicals in the plant, including other cannabinoids, terpenes and flavonoids. These liquids are often green from chlorophyll or honey colored and may have an unpleasant taste and smell. Some extraction techniques minimize the amounts of terpenes and chlorophylls in the tincture. Most tinctures and extracts are produced locally and do not meet the high level of consistency and quality control that come with large scale manufacturing organizations.

There are a handful of high quality, tested, certified contaminant-free CBD products available online or in stores around the country. Some of these brands include Absolute CBD, Isodiol, and Hemp Meds and Green Roads (see Photograph XII.) In addition, the website www.CBDoilreview.org provides up-to-date recommendations for high quality, available products.

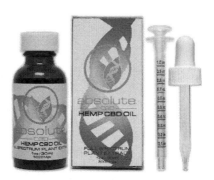

Photograph XII

Until cannabis was banned in 1937, pharmaceutical tinctures were the second most common medication available at pharmacies. It is interesting to note in states where medical cannabis has been legal the longest, the trend been away from smoked or vaporized cannabis and toward an increasing cannabis being sold as a tincture or edible. This is because of the perceived negative effects from smoking and associated social issues with the aroma of the smoked or vaporized medicine.

Tinctures and extracts do not work as quickly as smoked or vaporized medicine, but have a more rapid onset of action compared to other ingested forms of the medicine. The tincture is an approximately 75% alcohol vehicle that is delivered via a dropper under the tongue where more rapid absorption occurs via sublingual arteries. The drug misses much of the first-pass effect from the liver. Like smoked or vaporized medication, its effects come on quickly and dissipate rapidly in a few hours.

In addition, the precise measurements afforded by a dropper or oral syringe (see Photograph XII) and the precise concentrations of the tincture or extract, lead to consistent dosing for the patient. It is important to advise the patient not to swallow the preparation as this will cause it go through the GI tract to the liver and undergo the first-pass effect. If the tincture is added to a tea or liquid, then it absorbed as an "edible" form of the medication, with the slow and gradual onset of effect associated with all cannabinoids that go through the GI system.

The type of cannabinoids present (THC and/or CBD) and their concentrations will be documented on packaging. Like strains of cannabis, unless high quality brands are purchased these labels are often incorrect if the product does not have high standards of preparation, manufacturing and quality control.

Cannabis Butter and Edibles:

Cannabis butter, is a soft, light green, butter textured substance that is made from cooking the cannabis bud, with butter to extract the cannabinoids into the butter. It is seldom eaten by itself, but is used to cook and bake a wide variety of cannabis edibles.

In addition there are an increasing variety of candies, and flavored drinks that have extracted cannabinoids in them.

The cannabinoids are digested in the GI tract and go through the first pass effect of the liver. This means, that the time it takes to have an effect is much longer, about one to two hours, and that the effects last much longer, five to six hours. In addition, when THC is ingested and is metabolized by the liver it is actually converted to a different substance called 11-hydroxy-THC. This is many times more psychoactive than the delta-9-THC that is in inhaled cannabis. Whereas, approximately 85% of the CBD is metabolized into inactive compounds by the first pass effect, so ingesting (eating drinking) CBD is a less effective way to get medication.

Edibles and cannabis butter have several positive aspects. They have a slow onset of action, and prolonged duration or effect, making them good for chronic pain control, or nighttime dosing.

Edibles are hard to dose, because of the large variation in the batches of cannabis butter that is produced in small operations. Also, the amount of active ingredients in the edible decreases with longer duration of exposure to stomach acids. The presence or absence of food in the stomach can likewise affect absorption and clinical effects.

Eating too many milligrams of THC, not CBD, can cause dysphoria, a highly unpleasant sensation akin to agitation, panic, or impending doom. People will often go the emergency room when the dysphoria is very bad or prolonged. Be careful with edibles, especially when they are from small "mom and pop" manufacturers.

Like all products found in the dispensary, the amount of THC and CBD in the product may be incorrect due to problems with quality control, and manufacturing in small start-up companies making these edibles. Once again, when dosing and titrating start with a low dose, a small piece of the edible, and increase slowly, until you feel comfortable with the correct dose for the condition. Edibles can be hard to titrate because of the slow onset of action and long duration of effect. Often there is markedly less cannabinoid in the product than the label says. There are few standards for labeling and packaging for these products. A recent informal analysis of several popular brands of edibles in Colorado found only a minute fraction of the cannabinoid in almost all of the products sold by several manufacturers.

In time new regulations and enforcement will result in higher quality and standards for edibles. However, for the present time, the patient will have to become familiar with dosing different brands of edibles.

Patients like edibles, which like tinctures, do not require any smoke or vapor, and the associated tell-tale smell or respiratory tract irritation. They can be ingested anywhere. They are reasonably priced compared to cannabis bud or hashish.

A safety issue has been recognized with edibles that contain THC. They usually come is simple packaging, and they are usually tasty treats such as baked goods, candies or soft drinks. This has resulted in spike in the number of children mistakenly ingesting the edible and ending up in the emergency room. There are no reported deaths, but serious side effects from the euphoric effects have been reported. New laws are being enacted mandating packaging and requiring single wrap servings to prevent accidental excessive dosing. CBD only products, even in very high doses of hundreds of milligrams have no appreciable side effects or euphoria.

Below (Photograph XIII) is an image of an example label for a cannabis medication. In this case it is bud, and so it will show the amount of THC and CBD in percentage. It also shows that the product has passed a "Safety Screen," for microbes, fungi, and pesticides. If this label was on an extract, or edible it wouldn't have a percentage of THC and CBD, but would have the number of milligrams of CBD and THC per dose of serving.

Photograph XIII

Cannabaceutical™ Facts

Tested On: January 1, 2011

YOUR LOGO HERE — Blue Dream

Sativa Hyb.

14.20% Wt. Loss on Drying

		Safety Screen	
Δ⁹-THC Max:	13.6 %	Total Aerobic	GOLD
Δ⁹-THCA	14.9 %	Enterobacteria	SILVER
Δ⁹-THC	0.53 %	Yeast & Mold	BRONZE
CBD Max:	7.60 %	Pesticides	PASS
CBDA	8.12 %	Patients can visit
CBD	0.48 %	www.TheWercShop.com to
CBN:	0.25 %	learn more about this label and the test types reported.

CBD Infused Topical Medications

Hemp oil that is high in CBD is extracted and infused into a wide variety of vehicles, such as creams or lotions (water soluble), ointments or balms (fat soluble), sprays, lubricants, infused-rubbing alcohol or dermal patches that are applied to the skin.

Because the cannabis oils are fat soluble they don't penetrate very deeply into the tissues and tend to work just on the skin and in the tissue just under the skin.

Because there is little or no absorption of the cannabis into the bloodstream with topical preparations there are none of the side-effects, such as euphoria, anxiety, or addiction, that people worry about when using inhaled or ingested cannabis.

Cannabis-infused topicals have been used for hundreds of years, and have been shown to be particularly useful for a wide array of skin conditions, fibrotic conditions just under the skin, and locally inflamed or arthritis joints.

CBD Isolates versus Whole Plant Extracts:

The vast majority of CBD products available in stores or online are made with isolated CBD. This pure CBD has been extracted from the hemp oil and has only tiny amounts of the other cannabinoids and terpenes in the oil. The soon to be approved prescription medicine, Epidiolex(r) is one of these, it is 99% pure CBD oil. Usually these isolates are very clear, like that shown in photograph XIV. These pure isolates tend to have no smell or taste, since CBD is odorless and tasteless.

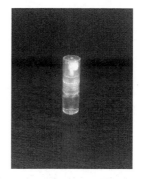

Photograph XIV

The preferred CBD products, however, are not isolates, but are made from whole plant extract. These extracts range from 3-20% CBD and the rest of the oil is non-THC cannabinoids, such as CBG, CBN, CBC, THCV and many terpenes. These whole plant extracts tend to be dark green and has a fruity or earthy flavors and aromas from the terpenes (see Photograph XII above.)

A 2015 study from Israel directly challenges one the main premises of the big pharmaceutical companies that artisanal botanical "whole plant" extracts are inherently inferior to pure isolates. The study was conducted by a one of the scientists who discovered the components of the ECS. The study showed that isolates of CBD have a "bell-shaped" curve when it comes to dosing. That is, as the dose of CBD goes higher, there is more of a therapeutic benefit. But at a certain dose, the effects actually become less. So, with isolates the goal is to find the "sweet spot" dose discussed in a later chapter. This need to find the "sweet spot" is not a good quality of a medicine, as there is only a narrow "window" for the correct dose, if the dose goes above that level, then the benefits rapidly decrease.

In the study they used a whole plant extract that was 17.9% CBD with tiny percentages of many other cannabinoids and terpenes. This is similar to Charlotte's Web and Absolute CBD extracts. They compared this in mice to an isolate of CBD, which was similar to Epidiolex(r). The whole plant extract had a direct dose dependent response to pain and inflammation. That is as the dose increased, so did the benefit. There was no drop off as the dose went higher. Of course, at a certain dose of CBD, there were no additional therapeutic benefits. This makes whole plant extract a preferable way to dose CBD. The researchers also found the a lower dose of CBD was needed to get the same benefits for pain or inflammation reduction. The researchers felt that the whole plant extract was a superior medication due to the "entourage effect" of the other cannabinoids and terpenes on the ECS receptors.

For this and other important reasons only whole plant extracts of CBD are recommended.

www.TheHempDepot.org

http://www.cwhemp.com

CHAPTER 4

HOW SAFE IS CBD

Cannabidiol (CBD) is very safe. It is essentially a plant oil, not unlike sunflower or olive oil. The main difference is that CBD interacts with ECS. It blocks an enzyme that ends up increasing the amount of our naturally produced cannabinoids in our body. So it is safe, and natural.

Hemp Oil

CBD is legal and available in all 50 states without a prescription only if it comes from low THC hemp plants, that were grown under the auspices of the 2014 Farm Bill. When it is extracted from these low THC cannabis or hemp plants it is considered by the federal government as a nutritional supplement that is 'generally recognized as safe' (GRAS) by the FDA.

Extraction techniques

There are several extraction techniques. Often, for the 99% pure CBD oil, the original hemp or cannabis oil has undergone four separate extraction techniques. The use of organic solvents such as butane and propane can leave behind a residue that is inhaled or ingested along with the CBD. It is recommended that only cold CO_2 extraction methods be used. But no matter what method is used, certified laboratories results of the marijuana bud, extract, or tincture should be available to the consumer, either online or at the dispensary.

Contaminants

There are no federal and very few and inconsistent state laws regarding testing for contamination of hemp or marijuana oil. In addition to the residues of organic solvents used to extract the oil from the plant material, there are several other significant contaminants to be concerned about. These include pesticides, heavy metals, microorganisms such as mold, and aflatoxins from fungi. Repeated low level exposure to any of these contaminants can have serious health effects. Again, the dispensary should have laboratory results that certify the absence of heavy metals, pesticides, microorganisms, and fungi.

CANNCON, Inc (www.jcanna.com) is a non-profit organization that was formed to provide high quality analytic testing to the medical cannabis community.

The educational website www.MedicalJane.com has a detailed analysis, by state of the current situation with getting accurate laboratory testing of medical cannabis, or CBD extracts, and tinctures.

www.medicaljane.com/2016/06/14/the-cannabis-contamination-conundrum

Consistency

Most high CBD cannabis bud, and CBD products will have significant variation in the potency from batch to batch. This is because cannabis is a plant, and the amount of CBD oil that it produces will naturally vary with different conditions. The CBD edibles, tinctures and other products tend to be manufactured by small companies and can also have issues with significant variation in the product. For CBD only products this is not a huge concern, because if one batch is slightly weaker than another, it will soon become apparent to the person using the medication and the dose can easily and safely adjusted. With THC, this is a different matter, because significant changes in the THC can have result in major side effects and euphoria, that do not occur with CBD only medication.

The few manufacturers of high quality CBD products test each batch for consistency and contaminants, when the oil is initially processed, and at the end of the manufacturing process. The also send batches of their products to independent laboratories for analysis.

Side-effects

There is some disagreement on the side effects of CBD. But this disagreement is only in patients using hundreds of milligrams of CBD daily, long term. This kind of dosing is only seen in severe epilepsy and neurologic disorders, where the CBD is being used under the care of a medical specialist to help decrease the other more toxic FDA approved medications.

For all intents and purposes in the dose ranges that are discussed in this book, 5mg to 400mg a day, there are no real side effects. There are some pleasant associated effects such as mood elevation, relief of anxiety, reduced inflammatory pain and stiffness from arthritis, and body relaxation. But none of these impair the brain, or one's ability to drive, think or operate devices or are associated with cancer or other chronic disease.

Allergy

Just like other weed pollen, such as ragweed, marijuana pollen may trigger an allergic reaction. There are hundreds of by-products in smoke that may trigger allergy. In addition, people may have an allergic reaction to contaminants such as mold, fungi and pesticides.

Although still uncommon, there are an increasing number of reports of allergy to marijuana bud and marijuana-based medications. The most common symptoms of allergy would be runny nose, nasal congestion, sneezing and a dry cough. Swelling and itching around the eyes, and hives on the skin have also been reported. There have been very rare reports of severe anaphylactic allergic reaction after eating a marijuana edible.

Some studies have suggested that exposure to hemp pollen in large outdoor grows, can result in people becoming allergic to marijuana pollen.

If you think that you are having allergic reactions to marijuana bud or extract, then you should discontinue using it, and discuss it with your medical professional.

Special Groups of People

As we have discussed CBD is exceptionally safe, essentially has no side effects, and can have significant health benefits for a wide variety of conditions. However, there are certain groups of people who should have focused discussion with their medical professional prior to considering taking CBD or cannabis products.

Pregnancy

Like most medications, there is very little research on the effects of CBD and THC during pregnancy. Approximately 2-5% of women report using marijuana during pregnancy. All of the marijuana oils are fat soluble and easily cross the placenta into the fetal blood supply. There are some animal studies that show that marijuana can affect fetal neurological development. One study in animals using very high doses of THC. that suggests that low birth weight and premature birth, and behavioral issues later in childhood. However, these were very high doses of THC.

This can be an issue, because THC has been shown to be particularly useful for the treatment of 'morning sickness', which occurs in 70-80% of pregnancy women. This is especially true when other FDA approved medications don't work or can't be used during pregnancy. One study from 1994, was done of Jamaican mothers. The mothers used a home-remedy of marijuana to treat the morning sickness. They were compared to similar Jamaican mothers who didn't use any marijuana. The study found no differences in birth weight, premature delivery or behaviors in infancy and childhood.

Three large studies of British, Australian and Dutch women did not find any association with marijuana use during pregnancy and low birth weight or premature delivery.

There are two ongoing studies of child who were exposed to marijuana while their mothers were pregnant. There is suggestion of increased behavioral issues, lower IQ and psychotic symptoms later in childhood. However, some of these effects may be due to the fact that the mothers also smoked and used alcohol during the pregnancy.

These studies are ongoing. More research on this topic needs to be done. Like smoking cigarettes, and drinking alcohol, the general advice is to refrain from using marijuana-based medication during pregnancy, or while they are actively trying to get pregnant.

Breast milk

All of the oils in marijuana are fat soluble, so small quantities will end up in mother's milk. Like most medications, there is very little research on the effects of CBD and THC on developing infants. One study All of the oils in marijuana can end up in the breast milk, as well as several of the metabolites of these oils.

One study suggests that daily use of marijuana by breastfeeding mothers could retard infant motor development. Another study found no effects on infants. These two studies both have problems, and more high quality research is needed in this area.

More studies are ongoing. More research on this topic needs to be done. Like smoking cigarettes, and drinking alcohol, the general advice is to refrain from using marijuana-based medication while breastfeeding.

Children

The brain continues to undergo important development up until age 25. The ECS in the brain is involved with laying down the correct nerve tracts in the brain. Excessive doses of THC have been shown in animals to affect the normal development of several nerve systems in the brain. There is some evidence in humans that regular use of THC, especially high levels or THC throughout the day can cause structural changes in the brain, which are associated with emotional and reasoning issues.

CBD, has most of its effects outside of the brain, in the body's immune system. However, CBD does cross over into the brain and there are effects in the immune system cells in the brain from CBD. CBD has been used in high doses in high quality randomized clinical trials for the treatment of intractable seizures in infants and toddlers. These studies of these infants do not reveal any significant side effects from CBD. Although, additional long term studies are needed.

Elderly

The elderly population will probably benefit the most from CBD. CBD has many positive effects on conditions that are common in the elderly, such as arthritis, dementia, and cancer. Unlike THC, which can cause many unpleasant side effects, such as anxiety, agitation, short-term memory loss, issues with balance and euphoria, CBD has none of these side effects. Because of the minimal side effects CBD is an excellent adjunct medication for elderly patients.

Because very elderly patients often don't metabolize medications the same way as younger adults, it is recommended to start doses at half the recommended dose and move the dose up gradually in very old patients.

Other medications

There are many medications that can interact with THC. Because THC has most of its effects in the brain, other medications that affect mood, balance, memory, or cause euphoria, can have synergistic effects when THC is also taken.

CBD, however, has almost no side effects. However, CBD and THC can inhibit the action of a very important enzyme system in the liver called P450. This enzyme system is involved with the metabolism and breakdown of 60% of the FDA approved medications that we use. There is a potential for slight increases in the blood levels of these medications with use of higher doses of CBD. For the vast majority of medications this slight increase is not important. However, for some drugs, such as anticoagulant and anti-epilepsy drugs this increase in blood level can have a serious effect.

Your medical professional can review which medications that you are taking and discuss using them in combination with CBD. Remember that vast majority of physicians and nurses have had no education about the ECS, THC or CBD. So, you may want to have them read this following excellent article on the subject of CBD and the P450 system at Project CBD.

www.projectcbd.org/article/cbd-drug-interactions-role-cytochrome-p450

Alcohol

Alcohol can cause euphoria, mood disturbances, balance and co-ordination uses, all of which can occur with THC. Alcohol used in high doses over a long period of time is associated with liver fibrosis and eventually potentially fatal cirrhosis. Once again CBD does not have these side effects. In fact CBD has been shown to decrease the brain degeneration associated with long-term alcoholism and reverse liver fibrosis in certain clinical situations. Studies in mice have shown that taking

CBD oil after binge drinking had a protective effect on the liver. It has been recommended to take 20mg of CBD as a preventative, however, further studies need to be conducted.

Drug Addiction and Dependencies

Persons with a history of drug/alcohol addiction or dependency are strongly cautioned against using THC. This because up to 9% of persons using high doses of THC, daily on a long-term basis may develop a dependency on THC. Being adolescent age, or having a history of other addictions greatly increases the likelihood of developing THC dependency. Fortunately, THC dependency is much more mild and easy to treat than other additions such as opioids or benzodiazepines.

CBD does not cause a dependency or addiction, so this is not an issues when using CBD.

Schizophrenia or Psychosis

Using high doses of THC has been associated with temporary episodes of paranoia and psychotic behavior. There is some research that shows an association between recreational THC use and the onset of schizophrenia. Because of this information, persons with a family history of psychosis or a prior history of a psychotic episode should not use THC.

CBD on the other hand has been shown to actually improve psychosis and is being evaluated for use as new type of anti-psychotic medication. Several promising studies in animals and humans have shown significant effects with schizophrenia and psychosis. It is not clear how CBD has these effects, but functional MRI studies of the brain have confirmed CBD has effects in the areas of the brain associated with psychosis. In addition, the temporary psychosis caused by excessive THC can be treated with one dose of pure CBD oil, 100-200mg.

CHAPTER 5

How to Use CBD?

Start low, go slow

Cannabidiol (CBD) is very safe, non-addictive and does not cause euphoria. THC has issues with addiction and euphoria, as well as several other issues with anxiety, agitation, coordination and short term memory. Because of all of the potential problems from THC, any time medical marijuana is used that contains levels of THC of 3% or greater, the medication needs to "start low" at a low dose, and gradually, "go slow", moving up the dose until the desired medical effect.

This is not the case with CBD only medications. In general there will be a recommended dose range, and you can start with this dose and increase as necessary based on the response. CBD is safe and without side-effects well into the 100mgs range. However, for most conditions that I discuss in this book, the treatment will be 100mg a day or less.

Sweet spot

When it comes to using THC or CBD for medical purposes, a little is better than a lot. Most of the therapeutic effects from THC and CBD occur in ranges of a few milligrams. If you take too much, the excess amounts of THC and CBD in the blood stream will literally flood the cannabinoid receptors (CB1 and CB2.) These receptors are not flooded naturally, so when this occurs, the receptors tend to sink inside the cell, leaving fewer receptors. This will result in more medication being necessary to get the same effect. When this occurs this it is called tolerance.

The goal when using THC or CBD is to get to the "sweet spot", the blood level that is high enough to have a therapeutic effect, but not too high that it floods the receptors and leads to tolerance. The recommended doses of CBD in this book are designed to reach these "sweet spot" levels in an average adult. However, it is expected that most people will have to gradually titrate up to the "sweet spot" dose, from the initial or starting dose.

Re-evaluate

After starting THC or CBD it is necessary to re-evaluate the condition to see if the dose of medication is having a desired and significant effect. Perhaps raising the dose a little will have more of a positive effect.

THC and CBD are not like aspirin or blood pressure pills, except for a few symptoms, you cannot expect a measurable effect until you have been taking the medication for several days. Generally, it is good to re-evaluate after the first two weeks, to see if the dose is working. Once you get to the dose that is working for you, then you can re-evaluate less frequently, such as every 3-6 months.

A diary is a good way to track the progress of your dose or medication. Document the dose taken, the time of day and changes in symptoms experienced. After two weeks you can look at the diary to get an idea of how the dose is working and make adjustments accordingly. There are several free or inexpensive apps for smartphones that have diaries for medical marijuana and symptoms.

https://www.sympleapp.com/

http://mypaindiary.com/

Tips on Dosing CBD:

Medical cannabis, which includes CBD, is unlike almost all other medications. First is it a plant extract that is often extracted and packaged without high levels of quality assurance. It can have contaminants such as left over pesticides, extraction chemicals, heavy metals from the soil, and microbes such as fungi. There are hundreds of CBD products on the market, but only a small number that address all of these quality and consistency issues. I recommend The Hemp Depot, Green Roads, or Charlotte's Web Hemp products, because they have independent testing and certification of good manufacturing practices to insure safety and consistency. In addition there products cost less or the same as inferior quality brands.

CBD is fat soluble, and therefore more difficult to absorb. Some brands are now making water-soluble CBD isolates, but these don't have the terpenes and may not have the entourage effect. Once CBD is absorbed most of it is metabolized before it ever gets a chance to have an effect. Because of this the best type of CBD medication is a full plant extract. This insures that the oil is in a natural balance with the terpenes and other cannabinoids.

As discussed earlier, the CBD can be inhaled, usually through a vaporizer, for quick but, short term effects, such as a flare-up of pain or spasm. For longer action, such as overnight, it can be absorbed by swishing on the inside of the mouth as discussed earlier. A few companies are now making suppositories (both vaginal and rectal) for specific conditions. Although there is little research behind using suppositories, there are plenty of persons who report benefit for menstrual cramping with vaginal CBD suppositories, and relief in inflammatory bowel diseases such as Crohn's disease, using rectal suppositories. The suppositories miss the "first pass" effect and probably deliver more medication to the source of problem.

Ingesting a CBD edible, or swallowing the CBD extract is not recommended. After the CBD is ingested in goes through the 'first pass' effect of the liver, and most of the active medication, is turned into inactive metabolites and excreted. Some available topical creams and patches purport to be effective in treating disease through the body, not just locally. However, because of the lack of high quality studies showing the absorption rates and efficacy at this time, none of these brands are recommended for effects, other than local application.

So although there are many ways to take your medicine, the most recommended way is to vaporize CBD for quick onset of action (10-20 minutes), and short duration of effect (60-90 minutes.) Swish the CBD around under you tounge for slower onset (30-45 minutes) but longer term effect (3-4 hours.)

Before starting treatment with CBD, start using a 'symptom diary'. There are several apps for your smartphone available to track how symptoms respond to medication. Find the right one, and start tracking the most important symptoms for a couple days, before you start the CBD. Based on what you read about CBD's effects on symptoms, later in this book, identify a handful of specific symptoms that you would like to see improved with the CBD. In addition to specific symptoms such as "sharp pain," or "stiff joints," you may also want to track your general 'mood.'

Each diagnosis in this book has a recommended 'Dosing' section. Unless there are reasons to start at a different dose, start at the recommended dose. Use the diary app to track how your symptoms respond over time to this initial dose. After four days at a specific dose, you will need to determine if you should increase the dose of stay at the current dose.

After four days of the same dose, you can decide if you want to increase your dose to get more of an effect. You can keep increasing CBD dose every four days until you feel that you are at the maximum effect. Remember that because of the "sweet spot" on the dose curve, if you start taking too high of a dose it will result in you getting lesser medical effects.

Typically you start at a specific dose, such as 10mg three times a day (that is 30mg total.) Then increase it by 5-10mg every four days, until you get to the "sweet spot" dose. Most of the conditions discussed in this book will respond to 30mg-400mg a day of CBD.

If you feel that you have had maximum benefit from the CBD dose, then just continue to take this dose on a long term basis. It is sometimes advisable to eventually taper off CBD. Many of the conditions that CBD treats might quiet down, or resolve, so that CBD is no longer necessary. If you are tapering of long term use of CBD, it would be advisable to cut the dose in half every four days, until you get back to the starting dose, then quit.

Work with a Medical Professsional

I have mentioned several times that your regular physician may have no knowledge or experience with using medical marijuana or CBD extract. If you can't convince your medical professional to help you add medical marijuana or CBD oil to your treatment, then you can find a compassionate, educated and experienced medical professional in your area at one of these three websites.

www.Leafly.com

www.MarijuanaDoctors.com

www.WeedMaps.com

The doctors that are listed at these websites have met certain criteria and are specialized in the use of THC, and CBD. Make certain that they are willing to communicate with your regular medical provider, so that your care and medication use is coordinated correctly.

Where to get CBD Medication

It is very important from whom you get your medication. Any medical marijuana products that contain THC will have to come from an approved dispensary. The staff at the dispensary are able to help you find the right type of medication, and method of taking the medication. In general, you will be able to buy one month of medical marijuana at a time. So each month when you go back you can discuss how the medical marijuana that they have recommended is working for you.

The following three websites list all of the state-approved dispensaries in your area.

www.Leafly.com

www.MarijuanaDoctors.com

www.WeedMaps.com

CBD oil is often bought online, as it is legal in all 50 states and able to be shipped across state lines. The important thing to remember is to select a high quality, contaminant-free product. There are dozens of websites selling CBD oil, but the vast majority of these are selling over-priced inferior products. Recently the FDA sent out 'cease and desist' warning letters to companies selling CBD oil and making health claims.

For several years now I have been asked by patients and doctors to recommend one brand of CBD product. Because of the issues discussed above, I have been very hesitant to do this. However, I have evaluated three companies manufacturing processes, laboratory testing, good manufacturing practices certification and products and I now feel very comfortable recommending the following three CBD manufacturers. Their products are available around the world in retail stores, and through online purchases.

Absolute CBD products

http://www.thehempdepot.org

http://www.greenroadsworld.com

www.CWhemp.com

The website www.CBDoilreview.org has some good information about many brands and CBD products. Also discounts on products are available through the website.

Drug Testing and CBD Use

A real and common concern among people using legal CBD products it whether it can cause of urine or hair drug test to become 'positive' for marijuana or THC. The answer is an emphatic 'no.' The tests that are conducted on hair and urine samples are very specific. They test for THC and metabolites of THC. CBD is an entirely different chemical and does not cross-react on the screening or confirmatory drug tests.

The real problem is buying a product that is supposed to have less than 0.3% THC in it, and actually buy one that has a lot higher concentration of THC. Using a product that is incorrectly labelled can and has resulted in a 'positive' drug test.

This is one more reason to only purchase CBD products that are from high quality manufacturers, such as The Hemp Depot and Green Roads, that have accurate labeling.

Getting Your Doctor Involved

Over 95% of doctors, pharmacists and nurses never learned about the ECS in school, and have little or no experience with CBD and medical cannabis. Instead of trying to educate your busy health care provider with a quick talk, I recommend you write down this website on a piece of paper and give it to the provider to look at when they have a moment. This is quick, concise, science-based discussion of the 'pros" and 'cons" of medical cannabis and CBD. In my experience, almost every provider will want to start learning more about the ECS, THC and CBD after looking at this convincing site.

"The 10-Minute Summary," at ProCon.org.

(http://medicalmarijuana.procon.org/view.resource.php?reso urceID=142)

SECTION II: CONDITIONS TREATED WITH CBD

CHAPTER 6

SEIZURES AND EPILEPSY

Personal story

A concerned mother of a child with epilepsy and autism came to see me. She was visiting from Georgia and wanted to get a medical marijuana card. She was going to use the card to get medical marijuana for her daughter and bring it back to Georgia. I examined her daughter and told her autism and epilepsy had a good chance of responding to CBD. I told her she didn't need a medical marijuana card. She could get all of the high quality CBD oil she needed, mailed right to her home in Atlanta. I gave her the name of a couple websites, including: http://www.thehempdepot.org, www.greenroadsworld.com, and the Charlotte's Web site. I told her, CBD oil was available without a prescription, and legally mailed right to her home.

She felt a little silly for driving seven hours each way to find that out, so I didn't charge her for the consultation. I told her to make certain that the Pediatrician in Atlanta was involved with her care. I got a nice email from her a few months later, and her daughter was doing great.

Introduction

A seizure happens when there are changes in the brain's electrical activity. Brain cells inhibit or excite other brain cells from sending messages and while there is usually a balance of these cells, during a seizure there is too much or too little activity, causing an imbalance. These imbalances can lead to chemical changes in the brain which cause a surge of electrical activity, resulting in the seizure. There are a variety of types of seizures including: non-epileptic, partial, and generalized. Non-epileptic seizures are usually caused by a head trauma and go away once the condition is treated. Some seizures result in little to mild symptoms, whereas severe seizures can lead to violent shaking and loss of control. As you can see for the "Symptoms" list, not all epileptic seizures result in dramatic movements of the arms and legs. Sometimes the seizure activity in the brain just results in an "aura" or sensation that something abnormal is happening, resulting in staring spells.

Epilepsy, is the diagnosis, when someone has a condition that results in recurrent seizures. Epilepsy or seizure disorder affects three million Americans. While any age group can be affected by epilepsy, the majority of new diagnoses are in children. It is a central nervous system condition in which nerve cell activity in the brain is disturbed, causing seizures. The causes of epilepsy vary and can include a specific problem in the brain causing the seizures, but more than half of epilepsy cases in children are idiopathic meaning they have no clear cause or obvious problem in the brain. There are several genetic causes of epilepsy, especially the very severe, intractable forms of infantile and childhood epilepsy.

To diagnose epilepsy a doctor will inquire about symptoms and may order tests like an EEG to measure electrical activity of the brain or an MRI to look at images of the brain. At this time here is no cure of epilepsy, only treatments. Medicine to prevent the seizures is usually the first treatment used to manage epilepsy, but a special diet or very rarely implantation of a nerve stimulator have also been used to treat the disorder.

Unfortunately in over 30% of the cases, even multiple prescription medications don't adequately control the seizures. In another significant proportion of the patients, the side-effects from the prescription medications are so bad that the patient can't take the medication.

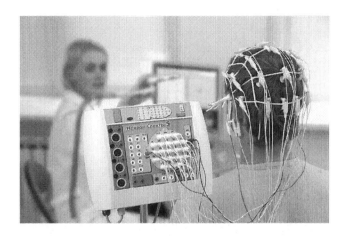

Example of an
Electroencephalogram (EEG)

Adult onset seizure disorder is usually due to head trauma, or other more clearly recognized conditions. However, just as many adults have problems maintaining control of their seizures with the available prescription medications.

The wide acceptance of the use of CBD for treating infantile seizures occurred after the Stanley Brother's began breeding a high-CBD strain of cannabis in 2009. This strain was eventually named "Charlotte's Web" in 2012 after Charlotte Figi had dramatic success with using CBD to control her intractable seizures. Subsequently the Realm of Caring (www.theROC.us) was started to provide assistance to these devastated families and children. I strongly recommend this website for anyone considering CBD or medical marijuana for their child with epilepsy. In addition to a patient-focused newsletter, they have local workshops and "care specialist consultations." They also have discounts for "Charlott'sWeb" CBD medications. The products from www.cwhemp.com have my highest reccomendation.

CBD Treatment

Epilepsy that has been found to be intractable, means that the medications are not controlling the epilepsy adequately. About 30% of children and adults diagnosed with epilepsy are not able to gain control of the seizures with the available FDA approved medications. Inherited conditions, such as Dravet's, usually cause intractable epilepsy, but many non-inherited causes of epilepsy are also unable to be controlled with up to 12 different FDA approved epilepsy drugs.

CBD has been shown to be somewhat to highly effective at significantly reducing frequency and severity of seizures. In a small study of treatment-resistant epileptic children, some of which had a specific condition and others who had idiopathic epilepsy, use of CBD was found to be effective in 16 of the 19 children. The average number of other drugs tried before the CBD treatment was 12. In this study 2 parents reported seizure freedom and 14 parents reported seizure reduction in their children. They also described other beneficial effects such as better mood, improved sleep, and increased alertness. These findings correlate with another major study at epilepsy treatment centers worldwide which showed that patients who received CBD treatment experienced a 45.1 percent reduction in seizures.

In a study done by Dr. Robert DeLorenzo his team found that cannabinoids decreased seizures by activating the brain's CB1 receptors. The "study indicates that cannabinoids may offer unique advantages in treating seizures compared with currently prescribed seizure medications... Ingredients in marijuana and the cannabinoid receptor protein produced naturally in the body to regulate the central nervous system and other bodily functions play a critical role in controlling spontaneous seizures in epilepsy."

It is clear that CBD has had positive effects on reducing seizures in children and adults with epilepsy, but this is a fairly new discovery with lots of room for further research and understanding of the relationship between CBD and epilepsy.

Autism spectrum disorder (ASD) has associated seizures in about 30% of the patients. The chapter on Autism discusses how CBD can help treat the functional symptoms of autism, and at the same time decrease the number and severity of seizures.

Epidiolex(r)

Epidiolex(r) is a patented pharmaceutical, manufactured by GW Pharmaceuticals. At the time that this book is being written it has had excellent results from high quality Phase III trials of the drug (www.GWpharm.com). It is 99% pure CBD whole plant extract from a patented strain of cannabis sativa. The biggest drawback of Epidiolex(r) and another GW Pharmaceutical extract, Sativex(r) is their extraordinary price, estimated to be $18,000-$30,000 a year for pediatric intractable infantile seizures. The similar 99% CBD extracts can be purchased online, and without a prescription at a more bearable cost of about $2000-$3600 a year.

Epidiolex(r) is very important because of the millions of dollars that went into doing high quality research in humans. These studies are reviewed at the Epilepsy Foundation website (www.Epilepsy.com.) The studied examined children with epilepsy that didn't respond to currently available medications, and showed that "seizures decreased by an average of 54%." Another study showed similar effects, but that 7% had some worsening of seizures with CBD.

Dosing

In general CBD has been shown to be helpful for long term control of the number and severity of the seizures. Because of this use a whole plant extract that is swished under the tounge. The starting dose is for children is ½ milligram per pound/weight, divided into three, equal, daily doses (morning, afternoon, and bedtime.) So a child weighing 100lbs would take approximately 17mg, three times a day, for a total of 50mg.) This dose can be doubled after four days to see if there is further improvement. Continue to increase by ½ milligram per pound, every four days.

So the second dose for a 100lb child would be 1mg per pound or 100mg, divided into three doses of 33mg each. Keep increasing until improvement plateaus. The maximum recommended dose is 5mg per pound a day.

THC, sometimes present in "High-CBD" products. can actually aggravate epilepsy, so make certain that the products you choose are certified laboratory tested, and have low amounts of THC (less than 0.3%).

Involving Medical Professionals

Childhood or adult-onset epilepsy is a significant and potentially life-threatening condition. Although it has not been reported, it is possible that the large doses of CBD required to control seizures to may change the liver enzymes metabolism of prescription drugs used to treat epilepsy.

Because of the complexity and severity of seizure disorder, and possibility medication interaction with CBD or medical marijuana, patients and guardians of patients with epilepsy should always work closely with their neurologist to determine if adding CBD or medical marijuana is appropriate. The neurologists, usually have little or no training on the subject and often won't actually recommend the CBD. However, then may give their permission to add CBD to the patient's treatment.

CHAPTER 7

HEADACHES AND MIGRAINES

Introduction:

Headache is a major public health concern, with enormous individual and societal costs. Each year about half of the population experience headache, including migraine (10%), tension-type headache (38%), and chronic daily headache (3%). Women are 2-3 times more likely to experience migraine and 1.25 times more likely to experience tension-type headache than men.

Migraine is the most common condition that medical cannabis has been used for in ancient and historical medical texts. A migraine is a specific type of vascular headache of varying intensity and is often accompanied by nausea, vomiting and sensitivity to light and sound. With more than three million US cases per year, migraines are considered common. The pain caused from migraines isn't usually caused by another disorder or disease. It is felt to be due to overactivation of the trigeminovascular nervous system that provides sensation to the face and head. Regular headaches are considered to be due to muscle tension, and present entirely differently from migraine.

Migraines affect people differently, with some people experiencing throbbing pain on just the right or left side of the head, and others experience pain all around the head. The pain can range from moderate to severe, but usually interferes with daily activity. Migraine pain can last for just a few hours or in some cases, last multiple days.

While there isn't an exact cause of migraines, researchers and doctors do have an understanding of migraine triggers. Some triggers include: hormonal changes in women, stress, drinks such as highly caffeinated or alcohol, sensory stimuli, certain food or food additives, medications, or changes in sleeping patterns.

Family history can also influence migraines; often they run in the family. Women are three times more likely than men to get migraines, and they tend to peak during a person's 30's.

Most of the symptoms of the throbbing headache, nausea, and avoidance of light or sound are due increased excitation of the trigeminovascular system, resulting in the dilated blood vessels, and neural inflammation. The subjective sensation of an 'aura' that often precedes a migraine, has been shown to be due to increased signaling with the neurotransmitter glutamate. CBD has been shown to reduce this signaling.

While there is no cure for migraines, there are many treatment options such as changing diet and certain medications such as pain relievers and triptans. There are a variety of home remedies and ideas for preventing, treating, and reducing the effect of migraines.

Studies have shown that persons who have migraine or chronic headaches are highly associated with other conditions such as anxiety, depression, chronic pain disorders and epilepsy.

<u>Migraine Symptoms</u>

Aura

Nausea

Light/sound sensitivity

Throbbing/pulsating pain

Vision changes

Pain on one side of head

Vomiting

Stiff neck

Dizziness

Weakness

CBD and Migraines:

Like fibromyalgia, and irritable bowel syndrome, Dr. Ethan Russo, one of the founding scientists of cannabinoid medications, feels that migraines are due to a deficiency of the body's natural cannabinoids. According to his theory increasing the body's level of natural cannabinoids by using CBD will reduce or other resolve the occurrence of migraines.

In a study done in Europe, researchers gave volunteers suffering from chronic migraines oral doses of a combination of THC and CBD. Once an oral dose of 400mg CBD/THC was administered, the acute pain caused by the migraines dropped by 55%. Phase two of the study found very similar results, finding that after three months, cannabinoids reduced pain among migraine patients by 43.5%. Some patients did experience drowsiness as a result of the oral dosage of THC/CBD, but otherwise the side effects were positive.

CBD can actually reduce to occurrence and severity of the episodes, so it is used as a preventive medicine. CBD is not generally used to control the acute onset of pain associated with migraines or non-migraine headaches

Doses for migraine and chronic tension-headache prevention

CBD Extract:

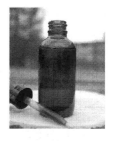

Starting adult dose (not recommended in children) 10mg of CBD extract under the tongue (oromuscosal absorption), morning, afternoon and bedtime.

May increase by 10mg every four days depending on response to the medication. Once maximum relief has been achieved with a certain dose, maintain that dose. Maximum daily dose 400mg.

CBD is not generally recommended for use for an acute headache or migraine. The slow onset of action of CBD and the lack of efficacy for acute pain, make CBD a poor choice for treating acute onset headaches and migraines. There are many safe and effective medications to treat acute onset headache and migraine pain.

Treatment doesn't always work

Medicine is an art, more than it is a science. Sometimes the recommended treatment doesn't work. It may not work because the dose wasn't correct, or it may not work because the underlying condition causing the symptoms is more severe than originally thought.

Start out with the recommended CBD extract dose. If the maximum doses of CBD extract isn't providing enough relief of cravings, it is time to go back to your physician for some advice.

Involving Medical Professionals:

Headaches can be serious or may represent a more serious underlying condition. Starting CBD for headache prevention should be considered only after discussion with your neurologist or primary care physician. As is unfortunately usually the case, most physicians will have very little knowledge of CBD, or medical marijuana, and their use with headache prevention. However, it is important to give your doctor the opportunity to assist you controlling your headaches. Do not attempt to suddenly decrease or discontinue your prescriptions medications. Involve your doctor, why you gradually titrate the dose of CBD to control your headaches.

If your regular doctor won't work with you to dose medical marijuana you can find a compassionate, experienced licensed clinician who will, in your area at the following websites:

www.Leafly.com

www.MarijuanaDoctors.com

www.WeedMaps.com

CHAPTER 8

CHRONIC PAIN

Introduction

Chronic pain is defined by doctors as any pain that lasts more than three months. It is unfortunately a rather common occurrence with more than 3 million US cases reported a year. While some chronic pain begins without a specific cause, many people experience it after an injury or due to a health condition such as arthritis, back problems, migraines, or infections. The symptoms and duration of pain varies from one patient to the next, and can range from mild to severe. Some pain is continuous while other pain comes and goes.

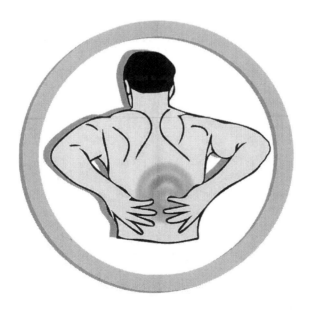

Back pain is a common
symptom of chronic pain

Mental health is often affected by chronic pain because it can take such a toll on daily life. Anger, depression, low-self esteem, anxiety, and frustration can all be caused by chronic pain. The depression caused by chronic pain can make the pain to feel worse, thus creating a cycle. While there is no cure for chronic pain there are a variety of treatments ranging from medication to acupuncture and lifestyle changes.

Chronic pain, can originate in the brain, nerves, muscles or at a site of trauma. Many patients with prolonged pain end up being prescribe addictive opioid medications, such as Vicodin(r), Lortab(r), Norco(r), Oxycontin(r), Diulaudid(r) and many others. The patient often ends up with both chronic pain, and a severe addiction to opioids, such that they perceive worsening of pain when the opioids are withdrawn. In addition to an intense opioid withdrawal syndrome. Secondly, long term use of opioids often results in depression, insomnia, and anxiety.

Types of Pain

There are several categories of pain, that are helpful in determining the correct treatment. Pain that originates at a site of injury such as an ankle sprain, or low back strain, is due to inflammation and swelling at the site of the injury. This causes achy, stiff, sore type pain. Over-the-counter topical analgesic creams, can include a combination of Capsaicin, Menthol, Camphor, Lidocaine and Salicylates. These creams are applied to the tender, swollen, injured area. These work by blocking the sensation of pain, while the injured tissue is healing. If the injured area continues to be swollen, tender or stiff for more than two weeks, than a topical version of CBD cream can be used. This stimulates the CB2 receptors to block release of the chemical messengers that are causing the inflammation and swelling.

If there is a large area that is injured or many areas, topical creams are not useful and an oral dose of CBD is usually helpful to decrease inflammation and swelling throughout the body. There is often beneficial anti-anxiety or mood effects from the oral CBD. Chronic pain can often be accompanied by anxiety or depression because of the effects of having chronic pain day after day.

When a nerve is irritated, pinched, or injured the nerve is damaged and this results in burning, sharp, shocking, tingling, radiating nerve pain messages, called neuropathy. These neuropathic pain messages are sent from the site of injury up to the brain, where they are perceived as pain. This is particularly common with diabetics, and people with herniated disks in the neck or back. When neuropathic pain becomes chronic, CBD can be tried. CBD can be used topically if it is a small area of pain, such as the soles of the feet. Likewise, it can be taken orally for effects in the brain, where is can reduce the pain messages coming up the spinal cord to the brain. This reduces the perception of pain, similar to the way opioids work. Other nutraceuticals, discussed below, are also very helpful for neuropathic pain.

Centrally mediated pain is dysfunctional pain that develops months after a painful injury or condition. It is a common problem in people with MS, Parkinson's disease, and brain or spinal cord injuries. It develops after the injured area has healed. It results in the perception of moderate to severe pain, without any underlying physical cause. Most patients who get started on long term opioids have this type central pain. Centrally mediated pain is similar to neuropathic pain with burning, sharp, or tingling pain. Often there are intolerable bursts of intense pain. This pain does not respond well to opioids, or most FDA approved pain medications. Several medicines used for depression or epilepsy have been shown to be useful to control this type of pain.

Unlike THC, CBD does not directly stimulate the CB1 receptors in the brain that have to do with pain perception. However, like anti-depressant medications CBD directly stimulate the serotonin receptors, resulting in an anti-depressant effect. It is through this same mechanism that anti-depressants such as Cymbalta(r), Celexa(r), Zoloft(r) or another class of antidepressants known as tri-cyclics, such as Amitriptyline, and Imipramine improve centrally mediated pain.

Fibromyalgia

Fibromyalgia is a common cause of debilitating chronic pain, often associated with insomnia, and depression. It is a form of centrally mediated pain, and several researchers have suggested that fibromyalgia may be due to a deficiency in the amount of naturally occurring cannabinoids in our brain. Reduced cannabinoids leads to a greatly increased perception of pain, such that even small pressure on a muscle will be perceived as painful in the brain. Likewise, decreased levels of the naturally occurring cannabinoids, ANA and 2-AG, result in insomnia, anxiety and depression. The goal of treating fibromyalgia then is to increase the cannabinoid tone in the brain. There is more detailed discussion in the chapter on Fibromyalgia.

CBD Treatment

CBD has been shown to be effective in managing symptoms of chronic pain in a couple different ways. It is thought that CBD interacts with receptors in the immune system and brain. These receptors are tiny proteins attached to cells that receive and aid in responding to chemical signals from different

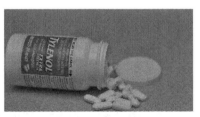

Tylenol is a common brand of acetaminophen

stimuli. When CBD interacts with these receptors it creates a pain-relieving and anti-inflammatory effect. This is similar to how medicines like steroid dose-packs, Aleve(r) and Ibuprofen(r) work. Often times chronic pain of the back or joints is caused by inflammation, and since CBD helps to reduce inflammation, pain patients have found that it aids in reducing inflammation and thus reduces pain.

CBD also works by modifying the perception of the pain in the brain. Such that the same level of pain is perceived as being lower. This is also how opioids work. Dr. Ethan Russo did a study and showed that cannabinoids proved to be 10-fold more potent than morphine in a wide range of neuron mediated pain.

Finally, CBD improves how well the opioids relieve pain, so that taking CBD at the same time as the opioid medication, results in the need for approximately 30% less opioid medication to achieve the same result.

For treating localized pain, inflammation, and swelling CBD topicals have proved to be effective. Topicals come in lotions, oils, or bath salts; some are infused with other plant extracts and create cooling effects like Tiger Balm(r) . Oils are good for specific stiff spots and bath salts relax and reduce inflammation while soaking in the tub.

When the pain is in more than just one or two specific places then CBD needs to be taken into the body via inhalation, mucosal membrane absorption of a spray or tincture or ingestion of extracts, gummies or edibles.

Other Pain Medications that Work with the ECS

Acetaminophen (Paracetamol), which is sold by the name Tylenol(r), is the most commonly used over-the-counter pain reliever. It is included in most opioid pills, such as Vicodin(r), Lortab(r), Norco(r) and OxyCodone(r). Usually 325mg of acetaminophen is added to each opioid pill for the synergistic effects. It is added to these opioids because it greatly increases the pain relieving effects of the opioids.

Acetaminophen has been around for 100 years, but it was only in the past decade that it was discovered how it relieves pain. Once the acetaminophen enters the body, it is metabolized by the liver into a drug called AM404. The AM404 blocks the uptake or the naturally occurring cannabinoid, anandamide (ANA). This results in increased CB1 activation by the increased levels of ANA. Activation of CB1 receptors results in turning down of the perception of pain in the brain. This is similar to the way opioids decrease the perception of pain. Because of this effect, acetaminophen can be used with CBD to have a separate effect on pain perception. CBD mostly decreases pain by decreasing swelling, inflammation and pain generation at the site of injury. Whereas, acetaminophen, reduces the perception of pain in the brain.

Palmitolethanolamide (PEA) is naturally occurring chemical in our bodies. It works with the ECS. It has been shown to be particularly effective of reducing neuropathic pain. Because it uses the ECS to work it is considered one of the cannabinoid medications, but is not found in *cannabis sativa*. PEA works differently than CBD, it stimulates receptors inside of the cells, and results in decreased swelling, inflammation and local pain generation at the site of injury. PEA is very safe, and is available as a nutritional supplement over-the-counter usually in 400mg capsules or bulk powder.

Dosing

In general, CBD is not recommended for acute or new onset pain. There are plenty of excellent, and safe over-the-counter oral and topical medications for treating strains, sprains, bruising, and spasm. If the condition persists longer than would be expected, then CBD can be tried. Topical CBD preparations are very effective for localized painful joints and muscles. If the pain is not localized then CBD extract swished under the tongue is beneficial. The starting dose is 10mg three times a day. This can be doubled every four days until it is maximally beneficial. Most painful conditions don't require doses above 100mg a day.

Remember that if something continues to be painful in the body, usually there is problem there, causing painful swelling, inflammation and sending pain messages to the brain. So it is not enough to just quiet the chronic pain, but the underlying cause of the persistent pain needs to be addressed. This best done by your primary care provider.

The WebMD website (http://www.webmd.com/pain-management/guide/pain-management-symptoms-types) has excellent advice and education about the possible causes of different types of chronic pain.

The dosing recommendations below also include advice on how to use PEA and acetaminophen.

There is a separate chapter on using CBD to taper off opioid medications and other addictive substances that are often used to treat chronic pain.

This dosing advice is for adults not using any other pain medications, or opioids. For advice on controlling chronic pain while using opioids, read the chapter of tapering off opioids with CBD.

Doses for Chronic muscle or joint pain/inflammation

Topical CBD balm:

Combine CBD balm with over-the-counter balm containing camphor, capsaicin, menthol and salicylic acid. Combine equal portions of the two balms and apply thin layer to the area using very firm pressure, morning, afternoon and bedtime. Deeply massage any knots or extremely tender points. Wash hands well after each application because the capsaicin

can burn mucous membranes. Do not apply near eyes, mouth or anus. Always read the directions with the packaging. Topicals can be used in combination with oral medication.

You can find a complete listing of all available over-the-counter topical balms containing camphor, capsaicin, menthol and salicylic acid at www.Drugs.com.

Doses for Centrally mediated pain or neuropathic pain in the extremities or localized area

Topical CBD balm:

Combine CBD balm with over-the-counter balm containing camphor, capsaicin, menthol and salicylic acid. Combine equal portions of the two balms and apply thin layer to the area using very firm pressure, morning, afternoon and bedtime. Deeply massage any knots or extremely tender points. Wash hands well after each application because the capsaicin can burn mucous membranes. Do not apply near eyes, mouth or anus. Always read the directions with the packaging. Topicals can be used in combination with oral medication.

PEA and acetaminophen can be taken at same times as CBD extract

PEA Capsule:

Starting adult dose (not recommended in children)400mg capsule once a day.

May increase after four days to 400mg twice a day, then up to three times a day, depending on response to the medication. Once maximum pain relief has been achieved with a certain dose, maintain that dose. Maximum daily dose 1400mg.

Acetaminophen:

Starting adult dose (not recommended in children). Prolonged or excessive use of acetaminophen can cause liver damage, and other conditions. This is especially true when using acetaminophen and alcoholic beverages. Always read the package insert and consult your physician if there is any question about the appropriate use of acetaminophen. Be careful to make certain that you are not getting acetaminophen (Tylenol(r)) in any other medications that you are taking.

625mg extended-release capsule three times a day. The extended release versions of Tylenol(r) is called "arthritis pain formula" it lasts eight hours and provides a more consistent control of chronic pain. This is the only dose recommended without consulting a physician. The maximum dose for acetaminophen is 3,000mg a day.

Doses for Fibromyalgia

CBD Extract:

Starting adult dose (not recommended in children) 10mg of CBD extract under the tongue, morning, afternoon and bedtime.

May increase by 10mg every four days depending on response to the medication. Once maximum pain relief has been achieved with a certain dose, maintain that dose. Maximum daily dose 400mg.

Treatment doesn't always work

Medicine is an art, more than it is a science. Sometimes the recommended treatment doesn't work. It may not work because the combination of medications wasn't correct, or it may not work because the underlying condition causing the pain is more severe than originally thought.

Start out with just CBD topicals and/or extract. If after 2 weeks you are not getting enough pain relief, add the acetaminophen. Give the acetaminophen at least a week to improve the pain. Finally add the PEA capsules. If the maximum doses of these three medications are not getting you enough pain relief, it is time to go back to your physician for some advice.

Involving Medical Professionals

In most cases of chronic pain, the original cause, a fracture, back strain, burn, etc. has healed. So the pain and the functional effects of the pain are the primary problem. As is unfortunately, usually the case, most physicians will have very little knowledge of CBD, PEA or medical marijuana, and their use in chronic pain. However, it is important to give your doctor the opportunity to assist you controlling your chronic pain. Do not attempt to suddenly decrease or discontinue your prescriptions medications. Involve your doctor, and ask her to help you gently taper off the prescription medications, why you gradually titrate the dose of CBD and other medications discussed above.

Sometimes CBD alone is not enough to get control of the pain and medical marijuana that has THC will be required. If your regular doctor won't work with you to dose medical marijuana you can find a compassionate, experienced licensed clinician who will, in your area at the following websites:

www.Leafly.com

www.MarijuanaDoctors.com

www.WeedMaps.com

Pertinent Website:

https://merryjane.com/news/here-s-how-cbd-can-help-ease-your-pain

Chronic Pain Support Groups.

https://www.fmcpaware.org/support-groups/browse-support-groups.html?sid=54:Support-Groups

https://theacpa.org/Support-Groups

https://chronic-pain.supportgroups.com/

CHAPTER 9

ADDICTION

Introduction

Addiction is considered a brain disorder characterized by compulsive engagement in rewarding stimuli, despite adverse consequences. It is a chronic disease of motivation, brain reward, and memory related circuitry. An individual with addiction pathologically pursues reward or relief by substance use or other behaviors. While there is a major focus on drug and alcohol addiction, addiction can come in many forms and affects millions of Americans daily.

The group called Sober Nation, explains addiction as follows:

'While the degrees of separation that exist between addiction and dependence can be can vague, those who display true addictive behaviors focus their energies on obtaining the substance or performing an activity to such an absolute degree they fail to meet their personal, social, familial, educational and professional responsibilities. Additionally, those who are in the grips of addiction act impulsively and even recklessly and will continue to engage in this pattern of behavior despite the consequences of their actions.'

When discussing addiction, the dopamine is often a point of discussion. Most addictions result, directly or indirectly, in the brain's reward system flooding the circuit with dopamine. Dopamine is a neurotransmitter, a chemical that transmits signals in the brain. It is present in areas of the brain that regulate movement, motivation, emotions, and feelings of pleasure. When a person's takes drugs, they can over stimulate this system, producing euphoric effects. These euphoric effects strongly reinforce the drug use behavior, causing a person to repeat the behavior.

What actually happens is the hippocampus (part of the brain involved with memory) lays down memories of this rapid sense of satisfaction, and the amygdala (part of the brain responsible for emotional responses) creates a conditioned response to the drug or behavior.

When a person repeatedly takes drugs or does an addictive behavior their brain begins to adjust to the overwhelming surges of dopamine by producing less or reducing the number of receptors that can receive dopamine signals. When this happens a person needs to keep taking more of the drugs or do the behavior more intensely in order to bring their dopamine function back up to normal. This is called tolerance.

There is no direct cause of addiction, but there are definitely risk factors such as genetic, environmental, psychological history, childhood history of abuse.

<u>Some Types of Addiction:</u>

Drug

Alcohol

Gambling

Sex

Shopping

Exercise

Internet

Pornography

Video Games

Nicotine

According to Narconon.org, an addicted person experiencing drug cravings will feel like life itself is dependent on getting and consuming whatever substance or doing whatever behavior is causing those cravings. They will feel justified in saying or doing whatever it takes to feel that satisfaction and relief."

Scientists have found that the symptoms of craving are mediated by increased transmission of the neurotransmitter, glutamate found in areas of the brain such as the hippocampus, the region in the brain responsible for learning and memory. This may explain why cravings such as anxiety, irritability, sweating and palpitations can occur years into abstinence, when a situation or person stimulates a drug related memory, creating a greater risk of relapse.

The concept of cannabis as a "gateway drug" has been debunked by the National Academies of Medicine in 1999. To the contrary, studies from Holland suggest that legal cannabis use actually decreased the likelihood of trying cocaine and amphetamines.

CBD Treatment

As was discussed earlier in the book, cannabinoid receptors are concentrated in several centers of the brain. One of those centers is the reward center, called the nucleus accumbens (ah-come-Ben's) Recent evidence has shown that CBD can reduce cravings and addictive behaviors, and reduce depression and improve mood, all which aid in addiction recovery.

The research has shown that CBD can reduce the occurrence of 'cue-induced cravings." This is a craving brought on by a specific trigger, such as craving a cigarette each time you get on the phone. Once again, we see CBD impacting health by modifying the response to a stored memory in the hippocampus.

Despite the different treatment options for opioid withdrawal, there still has not been a pharmacological treatment that has been proven completely effective in preventing relapse. Because of this fact, there is a "sense of urgency within the scientific community for the identification of new compounds that will help patients initiate abstinence and avoid relapse." Within this urgency of research the ECS and how it interacts with CBD and addiction has been a subject of increasing interest.

According to an article by Yasmin L. Hurd, *et al.* in various studies done with animals, CBD showed positive impacts on withdrawal symptoms. It consistently decreased stress vulnerability and improved performance in numerous animal models of cognitive impairment. CBD acted as an antidepressant and decreased compulsive behavior in rodents. It was shown to prevent cocaine-induced liver damage and lessen cardiac effects.

In a study of person quitting cigarette smoking, those using the CBD inhaler each time they craved a cigarette, found that they smoked 40% less cigarettes, compared to the placebo group where there was no change.

A recent study of young people with dependency on recreational cannabis/THC, showed that CBD is an effective tool to help with the cannabis craving. CBD actually is an antagonist of THC, and blocks the euphoric effects of THC.

In a recent study heroin addicts were administered a single dose of CBD over 3 consecutive days. Their propensity for craving was then tested by exposing them to opioid related triggers. The subjects taking CBD found their cravings were lessened, an effect that lasted for 7 days after treatment.

Some of the therapeutic benefit on CBD is also due improving the addict's mood and reducing anxiety. CBD's well documented effects of improving mood and reducing anxiety probably also contribute to its effects helping in addiction recovery. These effects are discussed in other chapters.

Doses for addiction and during withdrawal

CBD Extract:

Starting adult dose (not recommended in children) 10mg of CBD extract under the tongue (oromuscosal absorption), morning, afternoon and bedtime.

May increase by 10mg every four days depending on response to the medication. Once maximum craving relief has been achieved with a certain dose, maintain that dose. Maximum daily dose 400mg.

Treatment doesn't always work

Medicine is an art, more than it is a science. Sometimes the recommended treatment doesn't work. It may not work because the dose wasn't correct, or it may not work because the underlying condition causing the symptoms is more severe than originally thought.

Start out with the recommended CBD extract dose. If the maximum doses of CBD extract isn't providing enough relief of cravings, it is time to go back to your physician for some advice.

Involving Medical Professionals:

Addictions are serious conditions, and withdrawal from opioids and some other medications can have life-threatening sequelae. Starting withdrawal from a medication, drug or behavior using CBD should be considered only after discussion with your psychiatrist or primary care physician. As is unfortunately usually the case, most physicians will have very little knowledge of CBD, or medical marijuana, and their use in addiction. However, it is important to give your doctor the opportunity to assist you controlling your symptoms. Do not attempt to suddenly decrease or discontinue your prescriptions medications or illegally obtained drugs. Involve your doctor, why you gradually titrate the dose of CBD and use other addiction treatment services to control your condition.

If your regular doctor won't work with you to dose medical marijuana you can find a compassionate, experienced licensed clinician who will, in your area at the following websites:

www.Leafly.com

www.MarijuanaDoctors.com

www.WeedMaps.com

CHAPTER 10

USING CBD TO TAPER OFF OPIOIDS

Personal Story

Cynthia, a young mother, in her early 30's was a regular patient of mine. She injured her knee while skiing with her family over Christmas. I saw her originally and diagnosed a meniscal tear of the knee. I referred her to an Orthopedist for surgery. I didn't hear back from her after the surgery.

Several months later her husband came in to see me. He was tearful and depressed. He wanted to discuss starting an antidepressant. His wife had died from an unintentional opioid overdose. He told me that she had knee surgery and the surgeon has given her 90 tablets of Percocet for post-op pain. When she was in physical therapy the knee would flare-up and she kept taking Percocet. The surgeon was usually too busy, and the nurse practitioner would see her and kept refilling her Percocet.

After several months she realized that she was becoming dependent on the Percocet, and stopped taking it. However, she flared her knee up at work, and went back for more Percocet, after being off them for a month. She took about 8 tablets in one day and went into respiratory arrest and was found at home alone, dead.

This is unfortunately not an uncommon story. It is repeated 100+ times a day. But I have included it here because it provides some clarity to the real issues. Opioids are for short term use after significant injury or surgery. That's it. Within two weeks patients should be off all opioids and using other means to control the resolving pain unless you have late stage cancer. When you take potent opioids over time you will develop a tolerance to the drug, and have to increase the number of tablets that you are taking. In this case, Cynthia had stopped taking opioids for a month, so she was no longer tolerant to the high levels (8 pills a day) that she had been taking. So when she restarted opioids for a flare-up, and took her usual number of pills, she overdosed and died. Unintentionally. There are close to 100 of these unintentional deaths a day from doctor prescribed opioids! Unfortunately, there is little research to support long term use of opioids for this type of chronic non-cancer pain.

Introduction

Chronic pain has reached epidemic proportions in the past decade, with an estimated 80 million current chronic pain sufferers in the US. There has been concomitant exponential growth in the use of prescription opioids for chronic pain. There is an estimated 2 million addicted prescription opioid users in the US. A significant proportion of chronic pain patients are also being treated with dangerous anti-anxiety medications such as Xanax, and Klonopin. Much of this increase has been due to more loose physician prescribing habits fostered by aggressive pharmaceutical marketing campaigns. This increased use of addictive and potentially life-threatening medications has been associated with a four-fold increase in the number of deaths from prescription opioids between 1999 and 2015. The most recent CDC data estimates that 72 people a day die from prescription opioid overdose. There are over 700,000 opioids-related hospitalization annually. As many as two thirds of these deaths were in patients prescribed the opioids, who were not using drugs illicitly. One third of the persons who overdosed on prescriptions opioids were also taking a anti-anxiety medication. There is also a tendency to gradually increase dosage of opioids over time due to tolerance. Also periods of abstinence from opioids, due to problems obtaining opioids, may lead to unexpected overdose when the patient resumes the previous tolerated dose.

According to a 2016 TIME Health article, opioid and heroin addiction have become an epidemic in the past 15 years, and opioid addiction itself has accounted for approximately 59,000 deaths caused by overdose in America in 2016. The initial data suggest 2017 will be worse, and the president has officially designated it the opioid crisis as a "National Emergency." Opioids include drugs such as heroin, codeine, morphine, and pain relievers available legally by prescription such as oxycodone, Fentanyl(r) and Vicodin(r).

This epidemic of opioid prescriptions flies in the face of many studies that have found little evidence that opioids are effective treatment for chronic pain. Opioids undoubtedly help people with post-operative pain or after a broken bone. However, there are no high quality studies to show that opioids help long term, after the initial acute episode of pain. Another study found almost one million veterans found that 71% of patients who are started on opioids and maintained on them for at least 90 days, will still be taking opioids three years later. Unfortunately, physician prescribing practices are felt to be a major contributor to the opioid epidemic.

Chronic pain patients are commonly denied additional prescriptions for opioids due to failed urine drug testing, most often from marijuana (THC) that the person has obtained illicitly. These opioid addicted patients are suddenly without prescription opioids, and may seek out illicit opioids or much cheaper heroin. Due to accessibility and cost issues, these patients often end up using heroin off the street. This 'street heroin' is often cut with Fentanyl® and an even more potent elephant tranquilizer, greatly increasing the chance of fatal unintended overdose. An additional 26 people a day are dying from heroin overdoses.

There has been a public and political outcry to change the situation quickly and effectively. The efforts over the past few years have failed to significantly reverse the above statistics. The addition of medical cannabis or CBD, may be a significant part of the solution. Cannabis has been shown to have efficacy in opioid sparing, as an alternative analgesic, for mood elevation and to reducing opioid withdrawal and craving,

The CDC has recently released a report entitled "Prescribing opioids for Chronic Pain," that recommended "In general, do not prescribe opioids as the first-line treatment for chronic pain." This guideline excluded palliative or end-of-life care. It also recommended, "avoid concurrent opioid and benzodiazepine use whenever possible." Benzodiazepines, like opioids, are respiratory depressants. They work synergistically, opioids at receptors in the medulla oblongata and benzodiazepines as CNS depressants. The FDA has recently added a black box warning to address this.

In addition a more recent study added a new issue to the prescribed opioid epidemic. It showed dramatic increases in emergency room visits for unintentional overdoses of opioids in young children, and intentional use of family member's opioids in adolescents.

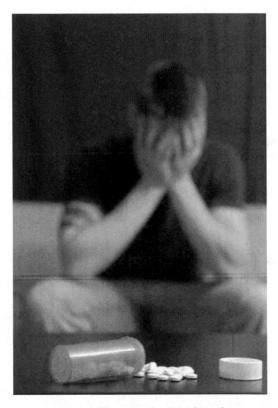

According to the National Institute on Drug Abuse, almost 100 people die everyday from drug overdoses.

Addiction is defined as a condition or disorder characterized by ingesting a substance or engaging in an activity that can be rewarding or pleasurable; the continuation of which become compulsive and has adverse consequences that interfere with ordinary life responsibilities, relationships, and health. Common substances in which a person becomes addicted include alcohol, nicotine, cocaine, and opioids. There is a separate chapter on using CBD for addictions. This chapter focuses specifically how to use CBD and other simple over-the-counter medications to gradually taper off of opioid medications and control pain at the same time.

Opioids are primarily prescribed to help relieve pain. They bind to opioid receptors on cells in the brain. By lowering the number of pain signals a body sends to the brain, they change how much pain the brain perceives. They can also affect the brain's pleasure system, causing a person to feel an addictive euphoric high. Several centers in the brain have opioid receptors and repeated use and abuse of an opioid can change the way a person's brain chemistry works. This change in brain chemistry can lead to psychological and physical dependence of the opioid. While opioids can be very useful for people recovering from serious injuries or surgery, they should only be taken exactly as prescribed and for only as long as necessary. Usually about a week or two.

When a person addicted to opioids stops taking them abruptly, they usually experience opioid withdrawal. This can occur simply in between doses of opioids, or when an individual stops taking the drug altogether. Depending on how dependent a person is on opioids, the withdrawal symptoms vary from mild to severe. Early withdrawal symptoms usually start within 30 hours for long-acting opiates like Fentanyl(r) and OxyContin(r) and within 6-12 hours for short-acting opiates, like Percocet(r) and Vicodin(r). Late withdrawal symptoms peak within 72 hours of stopping opiates and last a week or more.

This chart from the American
Addiction Center shows an
opiate withdrawal timeline

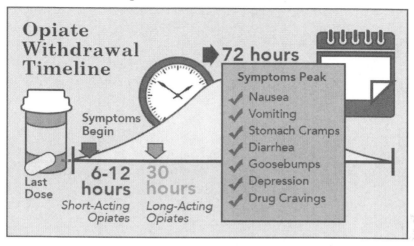

For those with opioid withdrawal there are a variety of treatment and detox options including medical detox which involves an individual being committed to a treatment center for 30 or more days and their vital signs being monitored. There is controversy about treating opioid withdrawal with another opioid medication, as some people view it as treating one addiction with another. There are also many treatment centers or "home-remedy" methods that take on a more natural approach treating withdrawal with diet changes, yoga, meditation, hydration, and natural supplements.

This chapter is not about withdrawing off opioids. Withdraw requires close medical supervision, excellent nursing, and use of several potent medications. This chapter is about gradually tapering down the opioid dose to reduce the hazards and side effects from the opioids. If this tapering is successful it can, over time, usually several months lead to the total discontinuation of the opioid medications.

CBD as an Adjunct Medication

CBD is not rewarding and does not induce drug-seeking behavior which are both characteristics of addictive substances.

CBD oil can be used as an adjunct medication for opioid sparing. Opioid sparing, means using another less hazardous medication to decrease or spare the amount of hazardous opioids that are used. Currently doctors use anti-inflammatory medications, antidepressants, anticonvulsants, and topical analgesic preparations, to reduce the amount of opioid necessary for adequate pain control. Opioid sparing, implies, that a lesser dose of opioid can be used to get the same effect, through synergistic effects of non-opioid medications.

CBD also has a positive impact on mood, anxiety, commonly associated with chronic pain syndromes. Also, CBD positively impacts inflammation, and spasm which often accompany chronic pain.

Decreasing the dose of opioids, via opioid sparing leads to fewer accidental overdoses, and less adverse effects such as severe constipation. A recently released analysis of the literature from the National Cannabis Industry Association (NCIA) discussed some promising observational and population-based findings supporting the use of CBD and medical cannabis as an adjunct to opioids and for tapering off opioids.

The primary objective of adding cannabinoid medication to chronic opioid therapy is to reduce morbidity and mortality associated with opioids, and improve function. The initial goal of opioid sparing, is to use CBD and over-the-counter acetaminophen safely to decrease the frequency of use and dose of fast acting opioids for breakthrough pain. The next goal is to gradually and safely reduce the dose and frequency of both slow and fast acting opioids for the baseline pain.

The goal of the initial phase of opioid sparing is to have the opioid patient learn to appreciate the ability to obtain symptom relief without any opioid, using the adjuncts of CBD, acetaminophen and other non-opioid medications. If these adjuncts are not providing enough pain relief, the patient then takes part or all the usual opioid dose if necessary. Over time, studies have shown, that a significant percentage of patient will spontaneously discontinue opioids altogether in lieu of CBD and other non-opioid medications.

A study of people using medical cannabis to taper off opioids showed that the common side-effects of chronic opioid use: constipation, depression, hypogonadism, and nausea were significantly reduced with concomitant use of cannabis.

Therapeutic effects of CBD

Cannabis has therapeutic effects on pain via the CB2 receptors. Stimulation of the CB2 receptors at the site of the pain or injury, results in decreased inflammation, swelling and decreased neuropathic burning pain sensation. CBD, like THC also improves the efficacy of opioids on the opioid receptors in the brain. CBD makes the opioid medication work better on the opioid receptor.

Other opioid sparing medications

Acetaminophen, also known as Tylenol(r), is one of the most commonly used over-the-counter pain medication. Unlike anti-inflammatory medications, and aspirin, acetaminophen has no gastrointestinal adverse effects or untoward cardiac or kidney effects. Acetaminophen is a common opioid sparing ingredient combined with opioids in several common prescription medications. 325mg of acetaminophen is added to a most of the opioid medications, including Vicodin(r), Lortab(r), and OxyCodone(r).

Acetaminophen has been used since it was invented one hundred years ago. However, how acetaminophen works was not discovered until the past decade. Once acetaminophen is ingested it is metabolized by the liver to a chemical called para-aminophenol, which works on pain by stimulating CB1 receptors. Para-aminophenol also an inhibitor of the uptake of the naturally occurring anandamide, leading to increased levels of this endocannabinoid and increased stimulation of CB1 receptors.

Para-aminophenol is also stimulates TRPV1 receptors, also known as the capsaicin receptors. TRPV1 is involved with providing to the sensation of heat, and sharp, burning pain.

CBD and Opioids Receptors

Opioid medications reduce pain by binding to and stimulating opioids receptors in the brain, leading to a decreased perception of pain via pain pathways that start in the spinal cord. CBD results in indirect amplification of the effects of opioids at the opioids receptor binding site. This effect is associated with observed synergistic effects of CBD and opioid medications.

Unfortunately, opioid receptors are heavily expressed on respiratory centers in the brainstem. Therefore, high doses of opioids can cause respiratory depression, the most common cause of opioid overdose death. There are essentially no cannabinoid receptors in the brainstem, which is the primary reason that no overdose deaths have ever been associated with cannabis use. However, although there are no fatalities associated with overdosing on cannabis, problems with decreased co-ordination have been associated with numerous cases of "death by accident."

How to Use Medical Cannabis for Opioid Sparing

The goal of opioid sparing, is to decrease the amount of opioid being used, while maintaining the same level of pain control. The motivation for opioid sparing includes reducing potential for life-threatening overdoses, decreasing the development of tolerance and escalation of opioid dosing and reducing serious adverse effects associated with long term use of high dose opioids.

The plan includes taking a dose of CBD prior to each opioid dose. When a fast-acting opioid is used, the patient will use fast acting vaporized CBD. When a slow release opioid is used, the patient will use CBD extract under the tongue, which comes on slowly.

For a vaporized CBD, take the recommended dose (see Flow Diagram below) then wait 15 minutes. The vaporized CBD will reach peak plasma concentrations in the blood in 9-23 minutes. If pain control is not sufficient, the patient will then take a second dose, again waiting 15 minutes to decide whether a before a fast-acting opioid is necessary. If there is measurable improvement in pain levels from the CBD alone, but not sufficient pain relief, then take half of the usual dose of the fast-acting opioid medication. For example, if the usual dose is Percocet 10/325mg, cut this in half which will give on 5mg of the active opioid ingredient, oxycodone. Less opioid will be necessary because of the synergistic effect of CBD on opioid receptors.

The process is similar for slow release CBD, under the tongue. These CBD extracts are used to spare the use of slow release opioids. The patient will take the dose discussed in the Flow Diagram below. Wait 30 minutes, because of the slower onset of action of the extract compared to vaporized CBD. If after 30 minutes there is not sufficient pain relief, then take half the usual dose of slow release opioid.

If after 4 days at this dose of CBD there was insufficient pain control increase the dose by 50%. Again, evaluate this dose for 4 days, before considering increasing the dose. This is part of the slow titration of dosing with which most people will quickly become comfortable.

Once pain reduction has been established with the use of CBD, the use of opioid pain medications can gradually be reduced, keeping in mind the potential for opioid withdrawal and the need for an established protocol for with your doctor for opioid weaning.

CBD works on CB2 receptors to reduce the inflammation at the site of injury and it enhances how opioids work on opioid receptors in the brain. Acetaminophen, is usually part of the opioid pill. The big pharmaceutical companies realize how effective acetaminophen in decreasing pain, and add 325mg to most of the opioid pills that are available. As discussed above, acetaminophen decreases the perception of pain in an entirely different way by using the ECS. It works by stimulating CB1 receptors in the brain, this decreases the perception of pain messages being sent from spinal cord to the brain.

The main issue with acetaminophen is that taking too much can be toxic to the liver. So the goal is to not take plain acetaminophen, if you are going to also take an opioid pill, since this will double the amount of acetaminophen.

I recommend the 650mg slow release version of acetaminophen called Tylenol Arthritis formula, which lasts 8 hours. The other versions of acetaminophen only last 4 - 6 hours.

The maximum daily dose of acetaminophen is 3,000mg. Each opioid pill contains 325mg and each Tylenol Arthitis formula tablet contains 650mg. Do not exceed a total of 3,000mg in one day.

The Flow Diagram shows how to substitute acetaminophen for opioid pills.

Discontinuing Opioids

Eventually stopping opioids altogether is another potential goal. In this scenario, the goal is to replace opioids with CBD, and possibly acetaminophen. Prior to attempting this goal, the patient should have satisfactorily gained the skills, experience and education necessary to use CBD for opioid sparing purposes. After they have been able to successfully reduce opioid doses, many patients may attempt to taper off opioids and benzodiazepines on their own, because of the pleasant mood elevation, relief from constipation, and reduction of several opioid adverse-effects. However, any tapering needs to be done in conjunction with the treating clinician to avoid serious and life-threatening opioid withdrawal or other adverse side effects.

Involving Medical Professionals

In most cases of chronic pain, the original cause, a fracture, back strain, burn, etc. has healed. So the pain and the functional effects of the pain are the primary problem. As is unfortunately, usually the case, most physicians will have very little knowledge of CBD, acetaminophen, PEA or medical marijuana, and their use in chronic pain. However, it is important to give your doctor the opportunity to assist you both controlling your chronic pain, and with tapering off of dangerous opioids and other medications such as Valium(r) or Xanax(r) that doctors commonly prescribe along with opioids for chronic pain.

Do not attempt to suddenly decrease or discontinue your prescriptions medications. Involve your doctor, and ask him to help you gently taper off the prescription medications, why you gradually titrate the dose of CBD.

Sometimes CBD alone is not enough to get control of the pain and medical marijuana with THC in it will be required. If your regular doctor won't work with you to dose medical marijuana you can find a compassionate, experienced licensed clinician who will, in your area at the following websites:

www.Leafly.com

www.MarijuanaDoctors.com

www.WeedMaps.com

People on long term use of opioids have are typically tapered off opioid medications at a certain predetermined rate that ranges from 20% to 50% per month. The medical provider, based on training, experience and recent research should discuss the taper rate, and expected quit date, usually from 2 to 10 months in the future. The medical provider will need to re-establish the Pain Contract with the patient, with the addition of CBD, and educate the patient on the proper use, dosing, safe storage, and awareness of adverse effects. The medical provider usually monitors the progress of the tapering with regular visits and review of a Pain diary.

FLOW DIAGRAM FOR USING CBD

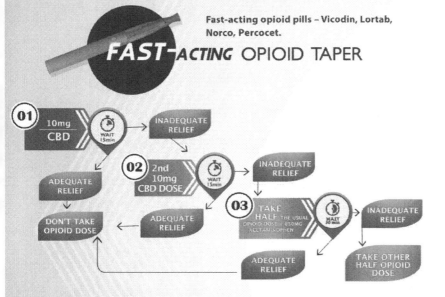

Fast-acting opioid pills – Vicodin, Lortab, Norco, Percocet.

FAST-ACTING OPIOID TAPER

01 10mg CBD → WAIT 15min → INADEQUATE RELIEF

ADEQUATE RELIEF

02 2nd 10mg CBD DOSE → WAIT 15min → INADEQUATE RELIEF

ADEQUATE RELIEF

DON'T TAKE OPIOID DOSE

03 TAKE HALF THE USUAL OPIOID DOSE + 650MG ACETAMINOPHEN → WAIT 20 min → INADEQUATE RELIEF

ADEQUATE RELIEF

TAKE OTHER HALF OPIOID DOSE

Both fast and slow release opioids can be tapered at the same time.

Cannabinoids are effective for all types of pain, centrally-mediated, neuropathic, myofascial, & sympathetically-medicated.

Most opioid tablets contain 325mg of Acetaminophen.

Prevention is better than treatment, limit use of opioids for acute pain to three day supply. Really need opioids for more than 2 weeks post-injury/surgery. Reduce to as needed dosing and lowest effective dose as soon as possible.

Set time frame, specific goals, tapering rate (20-50% per month)

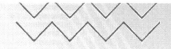

TO TAPER OFF OPIOIDS USED FOR CHRONIC PAIN

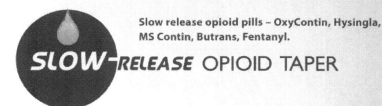

Slow release opioid pills – OxyContin, Hysingla, MS Contin, Butrans, Fentanyl.

SLOW-*RELEASE* OPIOID TAPER

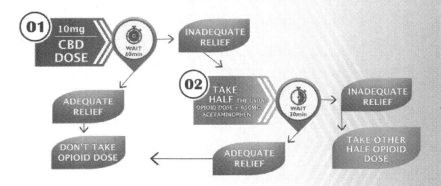

01 10mg **CBD DOSE** → **WAIT 60min** → INADEQUATE RELIEF

ADEQUATE RELIEF

DON'T TAKE OPIOID DOSE

02 TAKE **HALF** THE USUAL OPIOID DOSE + 650MG ACETAMINOPHEN → **WAIT 30min** → INADEQUATE RELIEF

TAKE OTHER HALF OPIOID DOSE

ADEQUATE RELIEF

Know the dangers of decreasing opioid tolerance & suddenly restarting medication at previous dosages.

Get your physician to prescribe some lower dosage opioid pills to help with the tapering process.

Use a "Pain diary" app to track long term progress more objectively.

Be educated about early signs of opioid withdrawal.

IF INSUFFICIENT PAIN RELIEF AFTER 4 DAYS, INCREASE DOSE TO 20MG THEN 30MG AFTER 4 MORE DAYS, & FINALLY 40MG AFTER 4 MORE DAYS.

CHAPTER 11

MULTIPLE SCLEROSIS, SPASM AND SPASTICITY

Personal Story

This one is a little different as I don't know the ending yet. But it is important nonetheless. A big guy named Brian, is a family friend. He has a very advanced case of MS and had been getting medical cannabis sent from a friend in California. He showed me his bottles of extracts, and said he wasn't noticing much effect and he was getting 'high' when he used the extract. The extract from California was very high in THC (20%) and had almost no CBD in it. Basically, the extract was made for getting 'high' and was certainly not for treating MS. I helped him get legal, safe, high quality CBD mailed to his house. He only recently got it so I can't tell you the effects, but in general MS patients love the effects on their burning pain, muscle and bladder spasms, and mood.

The important point is that just because it is from the marijuana plant, doesn't mean it's medicine. Most of the 'medical marijuana' for sale in California dispensaries is very high in THC and has almost no CBD. This is not going to treat anything but boredom. Get educated, know what you are buying, follow the dosing advice, and great things will happen.

Introduction

Multiple Sclerosis, abbreviated 'MS', is a disease in which the immune system eats away at the protective covering of nerves. This protective covering is called myelin. This myelin sheath, is similar to the plastic covering around copper wires. If the covering is removed the wire no longer transmits the electrical signal correctly. This nerve damage disrupts communication between the brain and the body, causing a variety of symptoms. While MS produces a variety of symptoms that impact each person differently, there are some more common symptoms as shown below.

<u>MS Symptoms</u>

Fatigue

Walking difficulties

Spasticity

Muscle spasms

Weakness

Numbness or tingling

Vision problems

Bladder/bowel problems

Pain

Cognitive changes

Depression

There is no known cause for MS and there are is also no specific test for the disease. However, there are often specific MRI findings seen in the brain or spinal cord. Doctors usually try to rule out other conditions that might cause the symptoms of MS. During the diagnosis process a person can expect blood tests, a spinal tap, a MRI, and a test which records electrical signals produced by the nervous system. While MS is not very common, it does affect more than 2.3 million people worldwide. It is thought that there are less than 200,000 cases a year in the

US, but because the CDC does not require physicians to report new cases and sometimes symptoms are invisible, these numbers are only an estimate.

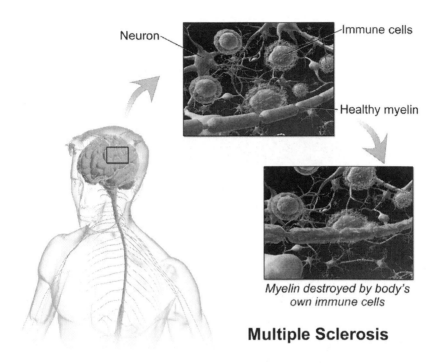

Myelin destroyed by body's own immune cells

Multiple Sclerosis

There is no cure for MS. Treatment is aimed at preventing progression of the attack on the myelin sheaths, managing the symptoms and speeding recovery from attacks. There are several treatments for MS attacks, corticosteroids which are prescribed to reduce nerve inflammation. Plasma exchange is another treatment options which involves removing the liquid portion of a person's blood (plasma) and separating it from the blood cells- the blood cells are then mixed with a protein and put back into the body. There is currently only one FDA approved medication, Ocrevus(r), which is used to slow the worsening of disability in people with primary-progressive MS. For people with relapsing-remitting MS there are many disease-modifying therapies used to attempt to treat the disease, but most of these options carry significant health risks. To treat the symptoms of MS physical therapy, muscle relaxants, and medications to treat fatigue, depression, and pain are commonly used.

Many people try alternative medicine as primary or as complementary treatment to help manage symptoms. Yoga, meditation, diet change, and exercise may boost overall physical and mental well-being, which in turn may provide some relief for MS symptoms.

CBD Treatment

Guidelines from the American Academy of Neurology recommend the use of oral cannabis extract for muscle spasticity and pain, but due to lack of research and evidence they don't recommend cannabis in any other form. Sativex(r) which is currently legal in 16 countries, although not yet in the US, is a mixture of THC and CBD with a 1:1 ratio and is administered as an oral spray. The drug is currently making its way through the FDA process, and once approved Sativex would be available in the US.

Researchers Vermersch and Trojano did a study with 281 patients who took Sativex for three months. After the 3 months MS and spasticity related symptoms such as: fatigue, pain, spasms bladder dysfunction and sleep quality were significantly improved. Patients also reported improved quality of daily living activities with the use of Sativex. Numerous other studies of the sort have been done producing the same results. It is not clear how much of these therapeutic benefits were from the THC versus the CBD.

In a study done by Italian researchers in 2015, they used only CBD topically. This study was conducted on mice with an experimental model of MS. The two main questions in this study were if a CBD topical affected the progression of the disease in mice and if the topical could recover paralysis of the legs? The researchers found "that use of the one percent CBD cream improved motor skills, including the reversal of back leg paralysis, a reduction in spinal cord damage, and a decrease in inflammation." While this was a small study done on mice, it provided interesting data that could eventually lead to the introduction of CBD in the treatment of MS. Human trials and more research need to be done to fully understand the relationship between CBD and MS, but studies such as this one provide insight in the benefits of CBD.

It is important to remember that researchers and doctors stress that CBD topical and alternative medicines such as Sativex(r) are only part of the therapeutic solution for sufferers of MS and similar diseases.

CBD impacts MS via several mechanisms. It decreases the autoimmune inflammatory destruction of the myelin sheath. This effect slows or stops the progression of the disease and decreases the symptoms or pain and spasticity (muscle stiffness.) CBD and THC both have positive effects on spasticity, through different mechanisms in the brain and body. CBD also has a positive effects of serotonin levels in the brain, improving sleep and depressed mood, both common issues with patients who have MS.

Dosing:

CBD Extract:

Starting adult dose (not recommended in children) 10mg of CBD extract under the tongue, morning, afternoon and bedtime.

May increase by 10mg every four days depending on response to the medication. Once maximum pain relief has been achieved with a certain dose, maintain that dose. Maximum daily dose 400mg.

Topical CBD balm can be applied to tight, or painful muscle areas three times daily.

Involving Medical Professionals

MS is a serious, and sometimes life-threatening condition. The medications that are prescribed for MS are also serious and need to be managed by a physician. Always involve your neurologist or treating physician with decisions to add CBD or medical cannabis to the treatment of MS.

Sometimes CBD alone is not enough to get control of the pain and medical marijuana that has THC will be required. If your regular doctor won't work with you to dose medical marijuana you can find a compassionate, experienced licensed clinician who will, in your area at the following websites:

www.Leafly.com

www.MarijuanaDoctors.com

www.WeedMaps.com

Pertinent website:

https://www.endoca.com/blog/news/new-hope-multiple-sclerosis-cannabidiol/

CHAPTER 12

FIBROMYALGIA

Introduction

Fibromyalgia (FM) is defined simply as chronic, widespread muscle tenderness and pain. It is a common disorder impacting more than 3 million Americans a year. This disorder affects more women than men, and can happen to anyone of any age. Just as with many pain disorders, symptoms can vary in type and intensity from person to person or even day to day.

FM Symptoms

Fatigue

Sleep disturbances

Cognitive difficulties

Stiffness

Depression

Anxiety

Tension headaches

Pelvic pain

Bowel/bladder issues

Migraines

While there is currently no exact cause of FM, decades of research is allowing medical researchers to begin to understand factors that might work together to cause it. Some of these possible factors include: infections, trauma, genetics, and stress. There are different thoughts on what causes the pain experienced with FM- one theory suggests that the brain might lower the pain threshold, changing one's perception of pain. Another thought is that the receptors and nerves in the body become more sensitive to stimulation, overacting and causing exaggerated pain.

FM is similar to MS in that there isn't a single test to detect FM, instead tests are done to rule out other potential causes of the pain and symptoms. Widespread pain for three months or longer, particularly pain that has no other identifiable cause, is usually the beginning of a FM diagnosis. Unfortunately FM is a chronic condition, meaning that the majority of people diagnosed with the disorder will have it the rest of their lives.

There is no cure for FM. Therefore doctors attempt to manage the pain and improve quality of life through medications. Pain relievers and antidepressants. Anti-seizure medications such as Neurontin(r) and Lyrica(r) are used because they stabilize nerves that send pain messages. There are alternative treatments for FM intended to be used in conjunction with medication these include: acupuncture, physical therapy, yoga, meditation, massage therapy, diet, and regular exercise.

CBD Treatment

There are have been various studies done on the relationship between cannabis and FM symptoms. One study of FM patients done by J. Fiz, *et al.* measured pain, stiffness, relaxation, and well being in 28 cannabis user and 28 non-cannabis users. The results found that after 2 hours of cannabis use, the users showed a statistically significant reduction of stiffness and pain, increased relaxation, and an increase feeling of well being. The conclusion of this study was that cannabis was associated with beneficial effects on some FM symptoms. It is not clear how much of the effects are due to THC versus CBD. Dr. Ethan Russo, one of the founding fathers of medical cannabis research, has postulated that FM is due to a deficiency of the body's endocannabinoids. Just like depression is due to a deficiency of the body's serotonin. Since CBD enhances the level of natural endocannabinoids in the brain and body, this treats the deficiency and reduces the body's response to painful stimuli. The elevated levels of natural cannabinoids also results in improved sleep and mood, both issues associated with FM.

Since FM is often accompanied by specific areas of the body that are very painful, both CBD oil taken orally, and topically applied CBD should be used.

In FM there is no actual injury or inflamed tissue or muscles. The problem is that the brain is perceiving pain throughout the body. So there is no need to actually treat any swelling or spasm. With FM the "tender points" around the body, are areas where slight pressure cause the sensation of unexpected or intense pain.

As we discussed above in the chronic pain chapter, PEA and acetaminophen are also helpful in reducing pain, or the need for muscle relaxants and addictive opioids.

Dosing

CBD Extract:

Starting adult dose (not recommended in children) 10mg of CBD extract under the tongue, morning, afternoon and bedtime.

May increase by 10mg every four days depending on response to the medication. Once maximum pain relief has been achieved with a certain dose, maintain that dose. Maximum daily dose 400mg.

PEA and acetaminophen can be taken at same times as CBD extract.

PEA Capsule:

Starting adult dose (not recommended in children) 400mg capsule once a day.

May increase after four days to 400mg twice a day, then up to three times a day, depending on response to the medication.

Once maximum pain relief has been achieved with a certain dose, maintain that dose. Maximum daily dose 1400mg.

Acetaminophen:

Starting adult dose (not recommended in children). Prolonged or excessive use of acetaminophen can cause liver damage, and other conditions. This is especially true when using acetaminophen and alcoholic beverages. Always read the package insert and consult your physician if there is any question about the appropriate use of acetaminophen. Be careful to make certain that you are not getting acetaminophen (Tylenol(r)) in any other medications that you are taking.

625mg extended-release capsule three times a day. The extended release versions of Tylenol(r) is called "arthritis pain formula" it last eight hours and provides a more consistent control of chronic pain- 3,000mg is maxium daily dose. This is the only dose recommended without consulting a physician.

Treatment doesn't always work

Medicine is an art, more than it is a science. Sometimes the recommended treatment doesn't work. It may not work because the combination of medications wasn't correct, or it may not work because the underlying condition causing the pain is more severe than originally thought.

Start out with just CBD topicals and/or extract. If after 2 weeks you are not getting enough pain relief, add the acetaminophen. Give the acetaminophen at least a week to improve the pain. Finally add the PEA capsules. If the maximum doses of these three medications are not getting you enough pain relief, it is time to go back to your physician for some advice.

Involving Medical Professionals

In patients with FM, there is no actual injury or inflammation in the muscles or tissues. The greatly increased perception of pain and the functional effects of the pain are the primary problem. As is unfortunately, usually the case, most physicians will have very little knowledge of CBD, PEA or medical marijuana, and their use in chronic pain. However, it is important to give your doctor the opportunity to assist you controlling your FM. Do not attempt to suddenly decrease or discontinue your prescriptions medications. Involve your doctor, and ask him to help you gently taper off the prescription medications, why you gradually titrate the dose of CBD and other medications discussed above.

Sometimes CBD alone is not enough to get control of the pain and medical marijuana that has THC will be required. If your regular doctor won't work with you to dose medical marijuana you can find a compassionate, experienced licensed clinician who will, in your area at the following websites:

www.Leafly.com

www.MarijuanaDoctors.com

www.WeedMaps.com

Pertinent website:

http://fedupwithfatigue.com/cbd-oil-and-fibromyalgia/

National Fibromyalgia and Chronic Pain Assocation - list of support groups:

https://www.fmcpaware.org/support-groups/browse-support-groups.html?sid=54:Support-Groups

CHAPTER 13

GASTROINTESTINAL CONDITIONS

Introduction

Colitis, Crohn's disease, Celiac disease, inflammatory bowel disease (IBD) and irritable bowel syndrome (IBS) are all disorders that affect the small and/or large intestine. It is important to understand the difference between colitis and Crohn's disease versus IBS. Colitis and Crohn's disease are considered inflammatory bowel diseases (IBD). Irritable bowel syndrome (IBS) does not fall into this category.

Relief of constipation was one of the original cannabis indictations cited in Shen-Nung, 5,000 years ago. Cannabinoids are anti-spasmotic relaxing smooth muscles. It helps with diarrhea by reducing inflamation in the intestinal wall.

Inflammatory Bowel Disease (IBD)

Colitis, which can be caused by infections or diseases including Crohn's disease, is an inflammation of the inner lining of the colon. The colon is a hollow muscular tube that processes waste products delivered from higher up in the small intestine. It also removes water and eliminates the remnants as feces. When a person has colitis or Crohn's disease the inner lining of this muscular tube becomes inflamed. Colitis is considered common with over 200,000 US cases a year. Whereas Crohn's disease, a specific type of autoimmune disease colitis, and is rarer. Colitis affects people of all ages, but the majority of cases are seen in people ages 18-60. The majority of Crohn's disease cases are seen in people ages 19-40. Both colitis and Crohn's disease patients are at increased risk for colon cancer and should be screened regularly by a physician. There is currently no cure for colitis or Crohn's disease and most treatments are focused on relieving symptoms.

Colitis Symptoms

Abdominal pain
Diarrhea
Bloody stool

Crohn's Disease Symptoms

Abdominal pain
Diarrhea
Weight loss
Fatigue
Anemia

Celiac Symptoms

Diarrhea
Bloating
Gas
Fatigue
Low Blood Count

Irritable Bowel Syndrome (IBS)

IBS is a an intestinal disorder that affects the colon causing various symptoms. Fortunately it does not put patients at higher risk for colon cancer.

There isn't a single known cause of IBS but it is thought that a variety of factors impact the disorder. Medical experts believe that some of the symptoms of IBS are caused by faulty communication between the brain and the intestinal tract. According to the Mayo Clinic the "walls of the intestines are lined with layers of muscle that contract and relax in a coordinated rhythm as they move food from your stomach through your intestinal tract to your rectum. If you have irritable bowel syndrome, the contractions may be stronger and last longer than normal, causing gas, bloating and diarrhea. Or the opposite may occur, with weak intestinal contractions slowing food passage and leading to hard, dry stools."

IBS is considered a common disorder with about 1 in 6 people in the US having symptoms at some time in there life. It also affects women twice as much as men, possibly due to hormonal changes in the menstrual cycle. While the disorder can affect people of all ages, it is most common in teen years through the 40's. There is currently no cure for IBS but through self-care and therapy, many patients are able to manage their symptoms. Changes in diet, exercise, and stress management can all reduce the severity of IBS and medications such as anti-diarrheals and laxatives may provide some symptoms relief.

<u>IBS Symptoms</u>

Abdomnial pain

Cramping

Bloated feeling

Gas

Constipation

Diarrhea

Mucus in the stool

The intestinal tract, including the small and large intestine, has high levels of CB2 receptors. Use of CBD that stimulates these receptors will result in a positive therapeutic benefit related to muscle contraction (colicky pain) and absorption of water in the stool (diarrhea or constipation.)

The high prevalence of CB2 receptors in the intestinal tract also means that CBD will turn down the inflammatory processes that cause colitis and Crohn's disease.

Like fibromyalgia, and migraine headaches, Dr. Ethan Russo, one of the founding scientists of cannabinoid medications, feels that IBS is due to a deficiency of the body's natural cannabinoids. According to his theory increasing the body's level of natural cannabinoids by using CBD will reduce or other resolve the symptoms of IBS. In the study he found that CBD demonstrated the ability to block gastrointestinal mechanisms that promote symptoms of IBS, celiac disease, and other related disorders.

CBD Treatment

Considering that there aren't any specific cures for colitis, Crohn's disease or IBS, research continues to be done on finding potential treatments for these conditions. Daniele De Filippis, *et al.* studied the effect of CBD on intestinal biopsies of patients with colitis and from intestinal segments of mice with intestinal inflammation. In the conclusion of their study they found:

"The results of the present study correlate and expand the findings suggesting CBD as a potent compound that is able to modulate experimental gut inflammation...in this study we demonstrate that during intestinal inflammation, CBD is able to control the inflammatory scenario and the subsequent intestinal apoptosis through the restoration of the altered glia-immune homeostasis. CBD is therefore regarded as a promising therapeutic agent that modulates the neuro-immune axis, which can be recognised as a new target in the treatment of inflammatory bowel disorders."

Colitis, Crohn's disease and IBS all involve inflammation or irregular muscle movements and issues with water absorption in the large intestine causing discomfort and a variety of symptoms. CBD increases the tone of the ECS. The gastrointestinal tract has large numbers of CB2 receptors. Activation of these CB2 receptors occurs through indirect effects of CBD. This reduces inflammation and causes muscle relaxation, providing relief of symptoms such as cramps, diarrhea, constipation, and spasms.

CBD rectal suppositories are absorbed directly into the bloodstream in the very vascular rectal area. The available information suggests that between 50-70% of the CBD is absorbed directly into the bloodstream from rectal 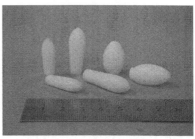 suppositories. This is far superior to the percent of CBD that is absorbed through the GI tract. The CBD does not go through the first-pass effect of the liver, and the CBD may also have more local effects in the colon that are not available from oromucosal absorption. For these reasons CBD rectal suppositories may be more effective than oromuscosal absorption. However, no research has been done to support the use of rectal suppositories over oromucosal absorption. Rectal suppositories only come in one dosage, 50mg. Therefore, it is difficult to gradual titrate a dose of a rectal suppository like you can with oil extracts. The price of suppositories is much higher per dose than using an extract. Certainly three times daily of insertion of a rectal suppository with a latex glove may not be an attractive option for many people.

Dosing

CBD Extract:

Starting adult dose (not recommended in children) 10mg of CBD extract under the tongue (oromuscosal absorption), morning, afternoon and bedtime.

May increase by 10mg every four days depending on response to the medication. Once maximum pain relief has been achieved with a certain dose, maintain that dose. Maximum daily dose 400mg.

If there is not optimal relief of symptoms with the 'maximum daily dose' then stop the oromucosal route and try using rectal suppositories (below.)

Rectal suppository:

Starting adult dose (not recommended for children) one suppository (50mg CBD) inserted into the rectum with a latex glove, morning, afternoon and bedtime.

Treatment doesn't always work

Medicine is an art, more than it is a science. Sometimes the recommended treatment doesn't work. It may not work because the combination of medications wasn't correct, or it may not work because the underlying condition causing the symptoms is more severe than originally thought.

Start out with just CBD extract. If the maximum doses of CBD extract and the rectal suppositories are not getting you enough relief, it is time to go back to your physician for some advice.

Involving Medical Professionals:

IBS and Celiac dsease are not life-threatening but can seriously impact a person's life. Trying CBD extract or suppositories to treat these conditions is generally very safe, and may be very effective. Colitis and Crohn's diseases are serious inflammatory conditions of the bowel and adding CBD should be considered only after discussion with your gastroenterologist or primary care physician. As is unfortunately usually the case, most physicians will have very little knowledge of CBD, or medical marijuana, and their use in colitis and Crohn's disease. However, it is important to give your doctor the opportunity to assist you controlling your colitis. Do not attempt to suddenly decrease or discontinue your prescriptions medications. Involve your doctor, why you gradually titrate the dose of CBD to control your condition.

If your regular doctor won't work with you to dose medical marijuana you can find a compassionate, experienced licensed clinician who will, in your area at the following websites:

www.Leafly.com

www.MarijuanaDoctors.com

www.WeedMaps.com

Pertinent website:

https://www.medicalmarijuana.com/medical-marijuana-treatments-cannabis-uses/cannabinoids-cbdthc-treat-symptoms-of-ibs/

CHAPTER 14

ARTHRITIS

Introduction

Arthritis is the inflammation of one or more joints, causing stiffness and pain in the tissues that surround the joints. According to the CDC more than 54 million American adults have some form of arthritis and about 32 million of those adults are of working age. It is important to note that arthritis does not refer to a single disease, but is an informal way of referring to joint pain or joint disease. There are currently more than 100 types of arthritis and similarly related conditions. Some more common types of arthritis include: degenerative, inflammatory, autoimmune, infectious, and metabolic.

Arthritis Symptoms

Pain

Stiffness

Reduced range of motion

Swelling

The symptoms caused by arthritis vary from person to person and even day by day. For some patients, arthritis symptoms may come and go and vary from mild to severe. For others, the symptoms may stay stable over a few years, or get worse over time. Not only is arthritis painful, but it can cause permanent joint changes and be so severe that the pain results in an inability to do daily activities.

The diagnosis of arthritis usually begins with a primary care physician to help determine the type of arthritis. If the arthritis is inflammatory or due to an autoimmune disease a rheumatologist, medical specialist in arthritis, is usually seen.

Depending on the severity of the arthritis sometimes orthopedic surgeons will do surgery such as joint replacements. There is currently no cure for arthritis and just as with the symptoms, there is a large variance in treatments used. Self care such as weight loss and exercise, therapies like massage and stretching, replacement surgeries, and medications such as anti-inflammatories, steroid and pain creams are all current treatments for arthritis.

CBD Treatment

As mentioned above, arthritis is characterized by inflammation of the joints. In a study done by Dr. Sheng-Ming Dai, it was found that CB2 receptors are found in unusually high levels in the joint tissue of arthritis patients. The use of cannabis is shown to fight inflammation in the joints by activating the pathways of CB2 receptors. These high levels of CB2 receptors are not present on healthy tissues, so the cells in the inflamed area results in increased production of CB2 receptors to help modify or reduce the local inflammation.

In another particular study conducted by A.M. Malfait, *et al.* they used mice with collagen-induced arthritis. The CBD was administered orally and injected into the mice after the onset of arthritis symptoms. They found that 5 mg/kg per day when injected and 25 mg/kg per day when taken orally produced the most optimal effect. The study concluded that CBD was effective in both the prevention of joint damage and the treatment of arthritis. When given to the mice orally it showed positive results, suggesting it is an attractive candidate for treatment of Rheumatoid arthritis (RA.)

Osteoarthritis is a type of arthritis characterized as a degenerative joint disease with cartilage degradation. Unfortunately right now there are no drugs or treatments to control the disease progression. However, there is increasing evidence that the endocannabinoid system (ECS) may be a therapeutic target for the pain created by osteoarthritis. In preclinical studies done with rodent models with osteoarthritis, there is evidence suggesting that the ECS plays a role in the functional changes of osteoarthritis. While there is limited clinical evidence at the moment, the preclinical studies indicate that cannabinoids such as CBD could play an important role in treating osteoarthritis symptoms.

There is quite a bit of evidence in animals showing that CBD is effective for arthritis. The Arthritis Society is currently funding grants for further research in the relationships between cannabinoids and arthritis and many other studies are being conducted on the topic, which will hopefully provide answers and relief for people suffering from arthritis.

There are several goals of treatment, to decrease the pain, decrease the swelling, stiffness and inflammation and finally to prevent the progression of the damage to the joints. The chapter on chronic pain provides a good discussion of how to use CBD, PEA and acetaminophen to treat chronic arthritic pain. Since CBD decreases the body's inflammatory response, it also results in decreased swelling, stiffness and inflammation of the joint. Finally, many cases of arthritis, such as RA and lupus are due to autoimmune conditions. When there is an autoimmune condition the body's immune system is attacking the normal cells in the lining of the joints. Since CBD modulates this autoimmune response, treatment can actually modify or prevent progression of the disease, and not just treat the symptoms.

The newer 'biologic drugs' advertised heavily on TV and long term use of steroid medications are associated with severe and sometime life-threatening side-effects. CBD by modulating the body's immune and inflammatory responses can result in your doctor decreasing or discontinuing these hazardous medications.

Some arthritis is limited to one joint, such as gout, or post-traumatic arthritis. Many times an arthritic condition causes joint swelling and pain in easy to reach areas such as the hands, knees or shoulders. In these cases, topical application of CBD balms in combination with over-the-counter creams containing camphor, salicyclate, menthol and capsaicin should be tried. The topical treatment can be tried by itself, or in combination with CBD extracts under the tongue.

Dosing for all forms of arthritis

CBD Extract:

Starting adult dose (not recommended in children) 10mg of CBD extract under the tongue, morning, afternoon and bedtime.

May increase by 10mg every four days depending on response to the medication. Once maximum pain relief has been achieved with a certain dose, maintain that dose. Maximum daily dose 400mg.

Topical CBD balm can be applied to swollen, painful joints three times daily.

Treatment doesn't always work

Medicine is an art, more than it is a science. Sometimes the recommended treatment doesn't work. It may not work because the combination of medications wasn't correct, or it may not work because the underlying condition causing the pain, swelling or stiffness is more severe than originally thought.

Start out with just CBD topicals and/or extract. If the maximum doses of CBD is not getting you enough symptom relief, it is time to go back to your physician for some advice.

Involving Medical Professionals

Arthritis can be a simple age or trauma-related chronic condition, or it can be a serious, and sometimes life-threatening condition. The medications that are prescribed for inflammatory forms of arthritis are also serious and need to be managed by a physician. Always involve your rheumatologist or treating physician with decisions to add CBD or medical cannabis to the treatment of arthritis.

Sometimes CBD alone is not enough to get control of the pain and medical marijuana that has THC will be required. If your regular doctor won't work with you to dose medical marijuana you can find a compassionate, experienced licensed clinician who will, in your area at the following websites:

www.Leafly.com

www.MarijuanaDoctors.com

www.WeedMaps.com

Pertinent website:

https://www.leafly.com/news/science-tech/the-medical-minute-can-cannabis-help-repair-arthritic-joints

CHAPTER 15

INSOMNIA

Introduction

A sleep disorder is defined as changes in sleep habits or patterns that negatively affect a person's health or function. There are many types of sleep disorders, two common ones being sleep apnea and insomnia. Insomnia is a disorder in which people have difficulty falling and/or staying asleep. Primary insomnia and secondary insomnia are the two main types of the disorder. Primary insomnia is when a person has sleep problems that are not correlated or caused by another problem or health condition. Secondary insomnia on the other hand, is caused by something else such as: depression, arthritis, cancer pain, or using a substance like drugs or alcohol.

Insomnia Symptoms

Waking up often during the night

Having trouble going back to sleep

Difficulty falling asleep

Waking up too early in the morning

Feeling tired upon waking

Irritability

Memory/concentration problems

It is thought that 1 in 4 people suffer from some kind of mild insomnia, and that most people will experience insomnia during their lifetime. For a health care provider to diagnose insomnia, they might do a few different things. A physical exam, a medical and sleep history, and possibly keeping a sleep diary for a week will help a healthcare provider better understand the insomnia. Sometimes people are referred to a sleep center where they undergo a sleep study either in a lab or with a machine at home.

There are many treatment options to aid in improving insomnia. Changing sleep habits, light therapy, and cognitive behavioral therapy are all non-medicated options to improve insomnia symptoms. A common treatment for insomnia is medications such as sleeping pills, but these can have unpleasant side effects. Many sleeping medications are addictive and can greatly increase the likelihood of an unexpected overdose of opioids, in those people using opioids for pain. Many sleep medications are not for dialy long term use, and may be addictive.

CBD Treatment

While there isn't a lot of clinically proven evidence out there regarding CBD and insomnia, there have been some studies done showing a potential benefit, but not in the way one might think. Unlike THC, CBD has been found to be mildly alerting at usual doses, rather than sedating. Numerous studies have been done with THC cannabis that have found cannabis as an effective treatment for insomnia. CBD, on the other hand, can still be effective in aiding in the treatment of insomnia, but in a different way than THC cannabis.

In a study done by Anthony N. Nicholas, MD, PHD, *et al.* they found that 15mg of THC proved to be sedative, while 15mg of CBD had alerting properties that actually increased wake activity during sleep and counteracted the sedative effect of the THC. This study, as well as a few others, found that CBD caused humans or rodents, to be alert, rather than sleepy. Therefore, it has been concluded that while CBD isn't an effective treatment for sleep disorders in terms falling and staying asleep, it is effective in reducing sleepiness and fatigue. A common symptom of people with sleep disorders is feeling tired throughout the day due to little or unrestful sleep; CBD can aid in treating this symptom by providing alertness and a feeling of energy throughout the day.

Separately, CBD has been shown to significantly reduce anxiety and feelings of "stress", this is discussed in detail in a later chapter. By reducing anxiety and perceived stress levels, people are often able to fall asleep more easily.

Dosing

Not recommended. CBD near bedtime can actually increase wakefulness. However, if perceived stress or anxious feelings are significantly contributing to the problems with falling asleep consider a trial of CBD an hour before bedtime. For more details see the chapter on 'Anxiety, PTSD and stress.'

CHAPTER 16

ANXIETY, PTSD, AND STRESS

Introduction

Anxiety is considered a mental health disorder that is characterized by feelings of worry, fear, nervousness, or unease. These mental symptoms are often associated with physical symptoms, such as rapid pulse, shallow rapid breathing, and dry mouth. These feelings are strong enough that they interfere with a person's daily life and activities. It is considered a common disorder with over 3 million cases a year, just in the US. "Anxiety" is considered a general term that includes different conditions, including panic, social anxiety, generalized anxiety disorder and phobias. In addition in this chapter we will discuss Post-Traumatic Stress Disorder (PTSD) and perceived "stress."

<u>Anxiety Symptoms</u>

Panic

Fear

Unease

Shortness of breath

Dry mouth

Sleep problems

Inability to stay calm or still

Tense muscles

Dizzines

PTSD Symptoms

Nightmares

Flashbacks

Avoidance of situations that bring back the trauma

Heightened reactivity to stimuli

Anxiety

Depressed mood

While researchers aren't sure exactly what causes anxiety disorders, a few things play a role. Environmental stress, changes in the brain, and genes can all be contributing factors. Anxiety disorders, like other mental health disorders, can run in families.

What all of these conditions have in common is that they are in response to 'adverse memories.' We store memories of a traumatic or emotional events in the hippocampus center in our brain. In most people these adverse memories gradually fade away. However, some people maintain the memory much more clearly, especially if it is at a very young age or particularly traumatic, such as occurs in war. When these adverse memories don't fade well, then the possibility of a recurrence of the adverse memory leads to the release of adrenaline, our "fight or flight" hormone. Adrenaline has developed evolutionarily to protect us in dangerous situations that our ancestors were dealing with on a daily basis, such as being eaten by a saber tooth tiger.

Once adrenaline is released into our body the blood rushes to our muscles from our organs to prepare to run away from danger or fight. This results in rapid heartbeat, rapid shallow breaths, dry mouth, trembling hands and often a feeling of impending doom. This is known physiologically as the "Stress Response," and works through a complex system that connects the emotional part of the brain to the body through the Hypothalamic-Pituitary-Adrenal (HPA) axis. When there is a true threat then this is helpful to our survival. However, in modern society this kind of danger is rare. Unfortunately, our brain and body have not evolved as fast as our society has changed.

So for many of us, the triggering of a simple adverse memory can result in an slight increase in our adrenaline release, giving us the typical symptoms of social anxiety disorder, or generalized anxiety. In others it may result in the release of a large amount of adrenaline, which results in the overwhelming symptoms of PTSD and some phobias, such as fear of heights or spiders.

The phrase "stressed out" or chronic stress, is not yet a true diagnosis. But represents what we feel when we are reminded of an adverse memory over a long period of time. Such as having a micro-manager boss, who is constantly checking up or criticizing an employee. This constant low level threat doesn't resolve, and leads to long term release of higher than necessary amounts of adrenaline. This long term release of unnecessary adrenaline, leads to increased release of our body's steroid hormone, cortisol, which is associated with elevated blood pressure, increased storage of fat, and reduced immune response.

There are no specific lab tests that can diagnose an anxiety disorder, but a medical doctor will ask questions about medical history, symptoms, and may do some tests to rule out other medical conditions. A doctor may then suggest a psychologist, psychiatrist, or mental health professional; these mental health specialists will ask questions and use tools and tests to find out more about the anxiety.

Treating anxiety disorders differs from person to person depending on their symptoms, medical history, and severity of the disorder. For some people self-care treatments such as: physical exercise, stress management, relaxation, avoiding alcohol, lessening caffeine, and having a healthy diet, are enough to treat the anxiety disorder so no further treatment is needed.

For others medications like antidepressants, anxiolytics, or sedatives are used to lessen the symptoms of anxiety. Cognitive behavior therapy, psychotherapy, and meditation have all proven to be helpful with anxiety disorders as well.

CBD Treatment

The hippocampus is one of the centers in the brain, it has to do with memory storage and memory processing. The hippocampus is also intimately involved with regulating the HPA axis, discussed above. The hippocampus has very high levels of cannabinoid receptors. Like several other centers in the brain, the hippocampus has an abundance of CB1 receptors. However, recent research has shown that there are also many CB2 receptors in the hippocampus. The new research shows that stimulation of these CB2 receptors raises the excitation threshold. What this means in practice, is that increased CB2 stimulation with CBD or other cannabinoid medications, decreases the responsiveness of the hippocampus to stored adverse memories. Since anxiety, perceived stress, and PTSD, are due to 'fear' of the recurrence of adverse memory, this results in decreased symptoms.

In a study done by researchers in Brazil, they found that CBD helped in treating anxiety disorders. They reviewed studies that used animal models, healthy volunteers, and people suffering from anxiety to conduct their research. In one particular study using mice, researchers investigated behaviors that were induced by fear caused by a snake in a maze. They found that the mice pre-treated with CBD, as compared to the non-treated control group, had significant reductions in defensive immobility and explosive flight. Even with these reductions, the mice treated with CBD showed no alteration in risk assessment and defensive attention. The results of this study provide evidence that CBD could be effective in the aid of panic attacks.

In the same review, the researchers found similar findings in human studies with CBD. Researchers conducted a study with the intent to investigate CBD and anxiolytic interaction using a group of healthy volunteers. The volunteers were asked to speak in front of a video camera for a few minutes, as public speaking induced anxiety in a lot of people. CBD, as well as diazepam and ipsapirone, was shown to significantly weaken the public speaking induced anxiety.

The conclusion of this review of studies involving CBD is as follows:

"Together, the results from laboratory animals, healthy volunteers, and patients with anxiety disorders support the proposition of CBD as a new drug with anxiolytic properties. Because it has no psychoactive effects and does not affect cognition; has an adequate safety profile, good tolerability, positive results in trials with humans, and a broad spectrum of pharmacological actions, CBD appears to be the cannabinoid compound that is closer to have its preliminary findings in anxiety translated into clinical practice."

Another study was done regarding CBD and anxiety, but this one focused on functional neuroimaging rather than self-assessment scales and physiological measures. In this study patients with social anxiety disorder (SAD), were given either 400mg of oral CBD or a placebo. Relative to the patients given a placebo, those given CBD showed significantly decreased anxiety and changes in the brain in association with lower anxiety. The researchers concluded that their results suggest that "CBD reduces anxiety in SAD and that this is related to its effect on activity in the limbic and paralimbic brain areas."

Hampson has shown that the anxiety-relieving effect of CBD can be blocked by a seratonin antagonist, indicating that this receptor is in part responsible for mediating the anxiolytic

effects of cannabidiol. Curiously, Hampson's current data suggests that in addition to binding directly to seratonin receptors, CBD may also act by altering the functionality of this receptor in such a way as to enhance its binding efficiency. In other words, CBD may actually magnify the effect of serotonin, in addition to directly activating the seratonin receptor.

Panic and THC

Panic, agitation and anxiety are all side-effects that can occur with some regularity in people who use cannabis. These side effects are due to the impact on the hippocampus and amygdala (emotional center in the brain) from high levels of THC. These side effects almost always occur with recreational use of cannabis. Too much THC, such as 20-30mg, in a short period of time, especially when there is very little CBD in the cannabis strain, often results in these unpleasant symptoms. These symptoms can be treated with 20-60mg of CBD oil under the tongue.

Medical-grade cannabis, are those strains used to treat medication conditions. Medical-grade cannabis has a ratio of CBD to THC of 1:1 or higher, which means there are equal or greater amounts of CBD in the cannabis, compared to the amounts of THC. For example, the cannabis strains to treat seizures are 20:1, with twenty times more CBD than THC. The strains used for most other medical conditions, and Sativex(r) spray is 1:1, with equal amounts of CBD and THC. These balanced medications, in usual doses, are not associated with anxiety, panic or agitation.

This book is only about CBD. CBD is not associated with any of these adverse side-effects.

Dosing for all prevention of all forms of anxiety, PTSD, panic and phobias

Long term daily use of CBD extract can have therapeutic effects on preventing and decreasing the symptoms of these conditions.

CBD Extract:

Starting adult dose (not recommended in children) 10mg of CBD extract under the tongue, morning, afternoon and bedtime.

May increase by 10mg every four days depending on response to the medication. Once maximum symptom relief has been achieved with a certain dose, maintain that dose. Maximum daily dose 400mg.

Treatment of acute or sudden onset of anxiety, PTSD, panic and phobias with CBD is not well studied. Other medications readily available through your doctor are likely to be much more beneficial, and have more rapid onset.

CBD Extract:

Sudden onset of symptoms, adult dose (not recommended in children) 20-60mg extract under the tongue immediately, one time.

Treatment doesn't always work

Medicine is an art, more than it is a science. Sometimes the recommended treatment doesn't work. It may not work because the dose wasn't correct, or it may not work because the underlying condition causing the symptoms is more severe than originally thought.

Start out with extract. If the maximum doses of CBD is not getting you enough symptom relief, it is time to go back to your physician for some advice.

Involving Medical Professionals

These anxiety and stress symptoms can be a serious, and sometimes represent deep psychiatric conditions. The medications that are for anxiety and stress-related symptoms and need to be managed by a physician. Always involve your psychiatrist or treating physician with decisions to add CBD or medical cannabis to the treatment of these conditions

Pertinent website:

http://www.healthline.com/health/cbd-for-anxiety#Overview1

CHAPTER 17

OBSESSIVE COMPULSIVE DISORDER

Introduction:

Obsessive Compulsive Disorder (OCD), is a chronic anxiety disorder characterized by excessive thoughts (obsessions) that lead to repetitive behaviors (compulsions). Obsessions are repeated urges, thoughts, or mental images that cause discomfort or anxiety. Compulsions are repetitive behaviors that a person with OCD feels the urge to do in response to obsessive thought.

Approximately 3.3 million Americans are afflicted with OCD, it usually starts puberty or late teens. An OCD individual usually experiences obsession over a particular thought such as the fear of germs; the compulsion in response would be to excessively clean or wash the hands. The compulsion is identified as unnecessary in the OCD sufferer, but anxiety over what will happen if they don't do the compulsive behavior generally makes the individual feel helpless to change either the thoughts or action that follows.

In most cases it is just an annoyance, but in some cases it can evolve into a condition debilitating to normal life. There are three common risk factors associated with OCD, as an exact cause is unknown. Genetics, brain structure and functioning, and a person's environment may all play a role in the chances of a person developing OCD. For example, people who have experience abuse or trauma during childhood are at an increased risk.

The severity of OCD varies from person to person, and severe cases can cause extreme distress and interfere with a person's daily life. Some people even develop a tic disorder such as motor movements or vocal tics. The symptoms of OCD can come and go, get better, and then get worse, or in some case are persistent throughout a person's life.

Diagnosis

While some people with OCD do notice their obsessive behaviors and compulsions, in most cases, particularly in children, the person does not realize their behavior is out of the ordinary. In children it is often parents or teachers who notice the OCD behaviors and bring it to the attention of a healthcare provider.

The signs and symptoms of OCD might be noticeable by oneself, but only a trained therapist can actually diagnose OCD.

Obsession Symptoms

Repeated unwanted ideas
Aggressive impulses
Fear of contamination
Images of hurting someone
Having things symmetrical or in perfect order

Compulsion Symptoms

Excessive cleaning/hand washing
Constant checking
Constant counting
Repeated counting
Repeated cleaning
Arranging items to face certain way

Treatment of OCD generally involves some form of antidepressants and anti-anxiety medications, as well as psychotherapy. The medications that are most effective are anti-depressants, that affect the serotonin neurotransmitter systems of the brain.

OCD affects each sufferer differently. It is not uncommon for patients with OCD to also have anxiety and depression. Cannabis is known to treat various forms of anxiety, and (CBD) in particular, has been shown in studies to have the potential to aid in the treatment of OCD.

CBD Treatment

While antidepressants provide relief for a lot of people, they do not come without side effects. Addiction, increased suicidal thoughts, loss of sexual desire, weight gain, and anxiety are all common side effects of antidepressants. Recently though, studies have been done showing that CBD is an alternative treatment for OCD without the psychoactive effects of THC and without the side effects of antidepressants. Another bonus being that relief from CBD occurs within days, whereas antidepressants can take many days or weeks to begin providing relief.

More importantly, CBD works by naturally balancing the endocannabinoid tone in the brain and body, resulting in healthier responses to 'adverse memories.' This results in improvement of OCD, anxiety and depression, which often occur at the same time.

There has not been much research in humans on the use of cannabinoid medications (THC and CBD) and OCD. However, based on what we know about how CBD works in the brain, it is likely that CBD results in decreased response to a fear of an adverse memory. This is how it helps people with anxiety, depression, and PTSD. By decreasing the level of 'fear' associated with not doing the compulsive behavior, the compulsion becomes less intense and more manageable. It is possible that CBD may also result in decreased obsessive thoughts as well.

Recent research has highlighted a positive outcome on the subject of the role that CBD could play in treating OCD. A study first published in October of 2013 in the journal, Fundamental & Clinical Pharmacology, by a team of Brazilian researchers investigated the effects of CBD on rats administered a chemical that leads to hormonal, physiological and behavioral effects; it is known to induce panic attacks and has been determined to worsen OCD symptoms. Later, the rats were given CBD in order to evaluate the obsessive-compulsive activity. The researchers concluded that the results of their study reinforce the anticompulsive effect of CBD.

The anticompulsive effects of CBD have been found to aid in reversing the obsessive and compulsive behaviors people with OCD experience. Researchers suggest this is due to the interaction between the sertonergic and cannabinoid system. Because CBD does not have any severe side effects it could potentially be an alternative treatment option for OCD patients who are experiencing negative affects from their current medications such as antidepressants.

Dosing

Long term daily use of CBD extract can have therapeutic effects on preventing and decreasing the symptoms of OCD, anxiety and lifting a person's mood.

CBD Extract:

Starting adult dose (not recommended in children) 10mg of CBD extract under the tongue, morning, afternoon and bedtime.

May increase by 10mg every four days depending on response to the medication. Once maximum symptom relief has been achieved with a certain dose, maintain that dose. Maximum daily dose 400mg.

Treatment of acute or sudden onset of OCD symptoms with CBD is not well studied. This should be considered a medical emergency. Other medications readily available through your doctor are likely to be much more beneficial, and have more rapid onset.

Treatment doesn't always work

Medicine is an art, more than it is a science. Sometimes the recommended treatment doesn't work. It may not work because the dose wasn't correct, or it may not work because the underlying condition causing the symptoms are more severe than originally thought.

Start out with extract. If the maximum doses of CBD is not getting you enough symptom relief, it is time to go back to your physician for some advice.

Involving Medical Professionals

OCD can be a serious psychiatric condition that can affect someone's social life and work. The medications for OCD need to be managed by a physician. Always involve your psychiatrist or treating physician with decisions to add CBD or medical cannabis to the treatment of these conditions.

CHAPTER 18

DEPRESSION AND MOOD

Introduction

Major Depressive Disorder (MDD), more commonly known as depression is defined by feelings of severe sadness, despondency and dejection. There are many types of depression of varying severities. Depression is a mental health disorder characterized by loss of interest in activities and a continually depressed mood, these feelings interrupt and impair daily life and activities. It is considered a common disorder with over 3 million cases per year in the US. There are different types of depression and while anyone of any age can suffer, women are twice as more likely than men to become depressed. Researchers also think that genetics may play a role in the likelihood of depression as it tends to run in families.

Depression Symptoms

Irritability

Persistent sadness

Fatigue

Loss of appetite

Difficulty with sleeping or oversleeping

Moving slowly

Thoughts/attempts of suicide

Aches and pains

A singular specific cause of depression is not known, but there are multiple theories on what the cause may be. One theory in particular that seems to be widely accepted is chemical function and brain structure alteration. Circuits within the brain that regulate moods might work less efficiently when someone is suffering from depression. Antidepressants, a common treatment for depression, are thought to improve communication between brain cells.

Types of Depression

Major Depreesion
Persistent Depressive Disorder
Bipolar Disorder
Seasonal Affective Disorder (SAD)
Psychotic Depression
Peripartum (Postpartum) Dissorder
Premenstrual Dysphoric Disorder
Situational Depression
Atypical Depression

A sad or depressed mood, is not a psychiatric condition. It is a natural response to loss. In general it is how our brain and body responds to a loss that results in an 'adverse memory.' We are sad over the memory of a loss. It could be the loss of a loved one, a job or money.

Sadness, such as a period of grieving, is a healthy response for navigating through life. The adverse memory usually fades over time. However, when this sadness or depressive symptoms last too long, become too deep or leads to self-destructive behaviors, then it is no longer healthy for us. This occurs when the adverse memory doesn't fade effectively.

As discussed in an earlier chapter on "anxiety and stress", the hippocampus is one of the centers in the brain, it has to do with memory storage and processing. The hippocampus has very high levels of cannabinoid receptors. Like several other centers in the brain, the hippocampus has an abundance of CB1 receptors. However, recent research has shown that there are also many CB2 receptors in the hippocampus. The new research shows that stimulation of these CB2 receptors raises the excitation threshold. What this means in practice, is that increased CB2 stimulation with CBD or some other cannabinoid medications, decreases the responsiveness of the hippocampus to stored adverse memories. Since sadness and depression are due to 'loss' associated with an adverse memory, this results in decreased symptoms of depression and an improved mood.

CBD Treatment

While antidepressants provide relief for a lot of people, they do not come without side effects. Addiction, increased suicidal thoughts, loss of sexual desire, weight gain, and anxiety are all common side effects of antidepressants. Recently though, studies have been done showing that CBD is an alternative treatment for depression without the psychoactive effects of THC and without the side effects of antidepressants. Another bonus being that relief from CBD occurs within days, whereas antidepressants can take many days or weeks to begin providing relief.

More importantly, CBD works by naturally balancing the endocannabinoid tone in the brain and body, resulting in healthier responses to 'adverse memories.' This results in improvement of both anxiety and depression, which often occur at the same time.

In a study done by Shoval G, *et al.* adult male rats (with the equivalent of human depression) were given CBD orally or were in a placebo group. Different tests were used with the rats to determine the effect of CBD. The results showed that CBD had a prohedonic effect on the rats treated; in a novel object exploration test and a locomotion test, CBD treated rats showed increased exploration and locomotion. The findings of this study express the beneficial effects CBD may have for the treatment of depression.

Depression and THC

Depression can be a side-effect with some regularity in people who use cannabis, especially in younger users. The side effect is due to the impact on the hippocampus and amygdala (emotional center in the brain) from high levels of THC. These side effects almost always occur with recreational use of cannabis. Too much and too frequent use of THC, usually observed in serious recreational users can cause a depressed mood.

Medical-grade cannabis, are those strains used to treat medication conditions. Medical-grade cannabis has a ratio of CBD to THC of 1:1 or higher, which means there are equal or greater amounts of CBD in the cannabis, compared to the amounts of THC. For example, the cannabis strains to treat seizures are 20:1, with twenty times more CBD than THC. The strains used for most other medical conditions, and Sativex(r) spray is 1:1, with equal amounts of CBD and THC oil. These balanced medications, in usual doses, are not associated with depression.

This book is only about CBD. CBD is not associated with any of these adverse side-effects.

Dosing for improved mood and depressive symptoms

Long term daily use of CBD extract can have therapeutic effects on preventing and decreasing the symptoms of depression and lifting a person's mood.

CBD Extract:

Starting adult dose (not recommended in children) 10mg of CBD extract under the tongue, morning, afternoon and bedtime.

May increase by 10mg every four days depending on response to the medication. Once maximum symptom relief has been achieved with a certain dose, maintain that dose. Maximum daily dose 400mg.

Treatment of acute or sudden onset of severe depression or suicidal thoughts with CBD is not well studied. This should be considered a medical emergency. Other medications readily available through your doctor are likely to be much more beneficial, and have more rapid onset.

Treatment doesn't always work

Medicine is an art, more than it is a science. Sometimes the recommended treatment doesn't work. It may not work because the dose wasn't correct, or it may not work because the underlying condition causing the symptoms are more severe than originally thought.

Start out with extract. If the maximum doses of CBD is not getting you enough symptom relief, it is time to go back to your physician for some advice.

Involving Medical Professionals

Depression can be a serious, and sometimes represent a life-threatening psychiatric conditions. The medications depression need to be managed by a physician. Always involve your psychiatrist or treating physician with decisions to add CBD or medical cannabis to the treatment of these conditions

Pertinent website:

http://thehempoilbenefits.com/cbd-for-depression

CHAPTER 19

PSYCHOSIS AND SCHIZOPHRENIA

Introduction

Schizophrenia and psychosis result in greatly disturbed thoughts, moods, and behaviors. There are many different forms of psychosis, some where the symptoms last only a few hours, and sometimes the psychosis lasts a lifetime. Schizophrenia, is an inherited condition, marked by the onset of psychosis in young adulthood.

Psychosis Symptoms

Depression
Difficulty concentrating
Suspiciousness
Delusions
Disorganized speech
Withdrawal from loved ones
Sleep troubles
Anxiety
Suicidal thoughts

Schizophrenia Symptoms

Thoughts/experiences that seem out of touch with reality
Disorganized speech or behavior
Decreased participating in daily activities
Memory/concentration difficulties

Symptoms vary greatly from person to person. Psychosis is a serious type of mental disorder characterized by thoughts and emotions that are so impaired it causes a disconnection from reality. Hallucinations and/or delusions are common characteristics of psychosis. These sudden onset of psychosis can be frightening for the person experiencing these thoughts, potentially causing them to hurt themselves or others. The causes and risk factors of psychosis are not completely known, but there are many theories. For example, certain illnesses such as Alzheimer's, Parkinson's, brain tumors, dementia, HIV that attacks the brain, and strokes have been shown to cause psychosis in some people. Other risk factors might include genetics, a family member with psychosis, or children born with a certain genetic mutation. Some types of psychosis can be brought on by specific circumstances such as drug and alcohol abuse or brief psychotic disorder, for example, can be brought on by extreme personal stress.

Hallucinations

-An experience involving the apparent perception of something not present

Delusions

-An idiosyncratic belief or impression that is firmly maintained despite being contradicted by what is generally accepted as reality or rational argument, typically a symptom of mental disorder

The current most attractive theory is that psychotic symptoms may be due to inflammation in certain centers of the brain. If this is true, then the ECS can have an important role in mediating the inflammation. However, this research is early and tenuous at this time.

CBD Treatment

Treating schizophrenia and chronic psychosis can be as varied as the different types and symptoms. Some treatments currently available include: medications, psychotherapy, hospital or residential programs, brain stimulation, or substance abuse treatment. These treatments have been shown to be successful in many cases, but unfortunately some of them, such as certain medications, have severe side effects.

CBD is a potential treatment option for certain types of psychosis. In numerous studies, CBD has been found to inhibit the episodic psychotic-like symptoms sometimes induced by THC. It has been shown to have antipsychotic effects, which is part of the reason it has potential as treatment or psychiatric conditions. In an online study done of over 1800 subjects, cannabis with a high CBD content was "associated with significantly lower degrees of psychotic symptoms, providing further support of the antipsychotic potential of cannabidiol". In another study done, specifically in relation to schizophrenia, the researchers concluded: "The anti-inflammatory and immunomodulatory effects of the non-intoxicating phytocannabinoid [CBD] are well established...Preliminary date reviewed in this paper suggest that CBD in combinations with a CB1 receptor neutral antagonist could not only augment the effects of antipsychotic drugs but also target the metabolic, inflammatory and stress-related components of the schizophrenia phenotype". Many other studies have found similar results. On the contrary, a study was done that found CBD was not particularly helpful in treatment-resistant schizophrenia, although it was not found harmful and the study only had three persons.

What these studies and research portray is that CBD definitely has antipsychotic effects that could be useful in treating psychiatric conditions. However, more research and clinical studies need to be done to find out more information and potential treatment plans.

Psychosis and THC

An temporary episode of psychosis can be a side-effect in people who use cannabis, especially with higher doses of THC and in younger users. These side effects almost always occur with recreational users of cannabis. Too much and too frequent use of THC in younger persons, especially if there is a family history or prior history of psychosis or schizophrenia.

There has been an ongoing and unresolved debate regarding THC causing schizophrenia. A review of the available evidence suggests that recreational use of THC, can uncover a person's predilection for eventually getting schizophrenia. That is, the person was already genetically at risk for eventually getting shizophrenia, and the use of high amounts of THC, seen in recreational use, uncovered the schizophrenia, earlier than it would have occurred, had they not used THC.

People with a prior history of an short psychotic episode, are at greatly increased risk for recurrent psychotic episodes with the use of THC, especially, large recreational amounts of THC.

Medical-grade cannabis, are those strains used to treat medication conditions. Medical-grade cannabis has a ratio of CBD to THC of 1:1 or higher, which means there are equal or greater amounts of CBD in the cannabis, compared to the amounts of THC. For example, the cannabis strains to treat seizures are 20:1, with twenty times more CBD than THC. The strains used for most other medical conditions, and Sativex(r) spray is 1:1, with equal amounts of CBD and THC. These balanced medications, in usual doses, are not associated with episodes of psychosis.

This book is only about CBD. CBD is not associated with any psychotic adverse side-effects.

Dosing

At this time the use of CBD for the long term treatment of schizophrenia or any psychotic condition is not recommended. Several significant studies are ongoing, to address the possible addition of CBD to treatment with other known anti-psychotic medications. This would only be done under the very close supervision of a psychiatrist.

Dosing for an acute episode of psychosis from too much cannabis/THC

There is enough basic science and clinical evidence to support the use of CBD to treat a single, acute episode of psychosis that was caused by use of cannabis/THC. CBD acts by antagonizing THC at the CB1 receptors, decreasing the effects of the THC.

CBD 20-60mg under the tongue one time.

Pertinent website:

http://www.medscape.com/viewarticle/839155_7

CHAPTER 20

NEURODEGENERATIVE DISEASE

Introduction

Alzheimer's, Parkinson's, and Huntington's are all neurodegenerative diseases. The dementia that occurs from repeated or severe head trauma is also a neurodegenerative condition. A neurodegenerative disease is characterized by progressive degeneration and/or death of nerve cells. Neurodegenerative diseases affect the neurons in the human brain, which are building blocks of the nervous system. Usually neurons don't replace or reproduce themselves, so when they become damaged by degeneration, it is usually permanent. As the disease progresses, problems with movement and mental functioning occur. Dementia is something caused by neurodegenerative diseases, such as Alzheimer's, and is responsible for the greatest burden associated with neurodegenerative diseases. Alzheimer's is a neurodegenerative disease with age as the greatest risk factor. The majority of people with Alzheimer's are over the age of 65, and the risk of developing the disease doubles every 5 years after the age of 65. Family history and genetics have also been found to be risk factors. Unfortunately age, family, and genetics can't be changed to help reduce the risk of developing Alzheimer's, but researchers are working on finding other factors that might be linked to Alzheimer's development which could be managed.

Neurodegenerative Disease Symptoms

Forgetfulness

Memory loss

Anxiety

Agitation

A loss of inhibition

Mood changes

Apathy

Tremors

Slowness of movement

Rigidity

While Alzheimer's mostly impacts the mental functioning of a person, Parkinson's affects the movement. Just as with Alzheimer's, Parkinson's generally affects people over the age of 60. Huntington's, is an inherited condition, it can affect people of any age, with most cases occurring around 30-50 years of age. Unfortunately as of now, there is no cure for these neurodegenerative diseases. There are some treatments to help manage the symptoms, but nothing yet that addresses the causes or progression of these diseases.

All of the neurodegenerative diseases mentioned above are caused by the destructive effects of misfolded proteins inside of nerve cells. Normal proteins are the bridges and transportation system inside of the cell. The proteins are shaped in specific patterns to function correctly for this transportation goal. The proteins can become misfolded due to various reasons (genetics, oxidative stress, toxins) and this can occur in different centers of the brain. When this occurs in one center it might cause issues with memory, and in another center it might cause a movement disorder.

These misfolded proteins don't work correctly and they accumulate like trash inside the nerve cell. The immune system uses various means to remove the damaged proteins from the nerve cells. Often as part of this removal process, the nerve cell is damaged. If the nerve cell is damaged repeatedly or severely it dies. This process of nerve destruction and death is very slow. It usually takes several decades from the onset of the disease until the first symptoms are obvious.

Underlying all of this is the immune system in the brain causing inflammation and gradual cell death.

CBD Treatment

As mentioned above, there is no cure for neurodegenerative diseases and research continues to be done by scientists and medical professionals to find a cure or treatments to help manage symptoms. There are many FDA approved medications for the symptoms of these neurodegenerative conditions, but none of the available medications actually slow down or stop the formation of the misfolded proteins or the immune system gradually killing nerve cells.

CBD and cannabis have been shown in several studies to be potentially beneficial in the treatment of some symptoms caused by neurodegenerative diseases, but also it can stop or greatly decrease the underlying disease process caused by the immune system.

CBD stimulates the CB2 receptors found on the immune system cells in the brain. This results in a decreased inflammatory response. So long term use of CBD would decrease the extent of damage caused by the inflammatory response.

THC stimulates the CB1 receptors found of the neurons, and this results in more decreased presence of these misfolded proteins through various cellular activities. Neurodegenerative conditions are best treated with a combination of CBD and THC.

In addition to halting or delaying the progress of neurodegenerative diseases, CBD also positively impacts many of the symptoms that are associated with some of these neurodegenerative diseases. As discussed in earlier chapters,

CBD can improve symptoms of tremor, spasm , depression, anxiety, and pain that can accompany some of these conditions.

Dosing for prevention and improvement of neurodegenerative conditions

Long term daily use of CBD extract can have therapeutic effects on preventing the onset, halting the progression and decreasing the symptoms of neurodegenerative conditions.

CBD Extract:

Adult dose (not recommended in children) 10mg of CBD extract under the tongue, morning, afternoon and bedtime.

These conditions are all very slow to progress and it may be difficult to judge response or progress without close observation by a caregiver.

Treatment Doesn't Always Work

Medicine is an art, more than it is a science. Sometimes the recommended treatment doesn't work. It may not work because the dose wasn't correct, or it may not work because the underlying condition causing the symptoms are more severe than originally thought.

Start out with the recommended dose, and give it 3-6 months to determine efficacy. If there is worsening of the condition, increasing the dose to 20mg three times a day is appropriate. Usually, it is not necessary to go to any higher dose because of the nature of this very slow, chronic disease process.

Involving Medical Professionals

Dementia, and neurodegenerative disease can cause serious, and sometimes life-threatening conditions. The medications need to be managed by a physician. Always involve your psychiatrist, neurologist or treating physician with decisions to add CBD or medical cannabis to the treatment of these conditions.

CHAPTER 21

CANCER

Introduction

As a generalized term cancer is a disease in which abnormal cells divide uncontrollably and destroy body tissue. The cells grow abnormally and have the potential to spread and invade other parts of the body. There are over 100 types of cancer that affect humans with the most common types in industrialized nations being: lung, breast, prostate, and colon/rectal. There are some general signs and symptoms of cancer, but it is important to remember that having some of these symptoms does not mean a person has cancer, as they could be caused by a variety of other conditions.

<u>Generalized Cancer Symptoms</u>

Unexplained weight loss

Fatigue

Pain

Fever

Skin changes

Change in bowel/bladder function

Non-healing sores

White patches inside mouth

Indigestion/trouble swallowing

Thickening or lump in body

Nagging cough

Cancer is considered one of the leading causes of death worldwide, with over 12 million people each year discovering they have cancer and over 7 million people dying from cancer each year. Unfortunately it is thought that over 300,000 cases of cancer each year in the US could be prevented through healthier lifestyle choices such as diet, exercise, and quitting smoking.

The treatments for cancer are just as variable as the types of cancer. The most common treatments include medication, surgery, chemotherapy, radiation therapy, targeted therapy, immunotherapy, and hormone therapy. Unfortunately these treatments for cancer can be intensive and may cause some serious side effects.

CBD Treatment

Both CBD and THC impact cancer through several important mechanisms. They increase cell death of cancer cells, through a mechanism of programmed cell suicide, known as apoptosis (a-pop-toe-sis.) All cells have the ability to commit suicide, and do this all of the time due to certain triggers. In the case of CBD and THC, this triggers a series of intracellular events only in cells that are rapidly dividing (cancer and tumor cells) resulting in apoptosis and cell death. It is not clear in how many types of cancers this occurs. However, it appears to work in breast, prostate, lung, colon and certain brain cancers.

Angiogenesis is the formation of new blood vessels (arteries and veins.) Cancers promote angiogenesis through various mechanisms to help it grow larger in size and get the oxygen and nutrients it needs. Therefore a lot of cancer research has been focused on anti-angiogenesis treatments. In a study done by M Solinas *et al.* they researched the relationship between CBD and angiogenesis. There results showed that CBD inhibits angiogenesis by multiple mechanisms. Therefore they concluded that CBD is a potential effective agent in cancer therapy.

Cancers don't just grow in size, they cause most of their damage by spreading throughout the body and growing new tumors in remote areas of the body. This process is known as metastasis (met-ass-ta-sis.) CBD and THC fight cancer by reducing the cancers ability to migrate, adhere, and invade tissue. This results in decreased proliferation and decreased metastasis to other parts of the body.

Other studies and research have found similar results in CBD's potential benefit of cancer treatment. Ligresti *et al.* showed in 2006 that CBD selectively and potently inhibited the growth of different breast tumour cell lines.

After a study done by Massi *et al.* it was concluded that:

'Collectively, the non-psychoactive plant-derived cannabinoid CBD exhibits pro-apoptotic and anti-proliferative actions in different types of tumours... On the basis of these results, evidence is emerging to suggest that CBD is a potent inhibitor of both cancer growth and spread.'

Not only is CBD showing potential benefits for anti-angiogenesis, but in some studies has shown potential in moderating inflammation and reducing the ability of some types of tumor cells to reproduce. Also as mentioned in previous chapters, CBD has been shown to have a positive effect on pain management, mood, fatigue, and bowel function. These are all possible symptoms associated with having cancer that may be alleviated by the use of CBD. However, CBD does not increase the appetite. The increased appetite and decreased nausea/vomiting effects associated with cannabis, are from THC.

Rick Simpson Oil (RSO)

Rick Simpson Oil (RSO) also known as Phoenix Tears is not to be confused with the high CBD hemp oil sold as Real Scientific Hemp Oil (RSHO). RSO, is a very potent form of thick green/black oil high in THC. It used at extremely high doses of 1000mg a day of THC for 60-90 days to treat late stage cancer. There are many case studies and anecdotal reports of it being effective for cancer. There are several information videos on Youtube about how to use this potentially life-saving oil.

RSO or Phoenix Tears which contain huge amounts of THC and are very challenging to use without education, counseling and guidance.

In addition the website -

www.CureYourOwnCancer.org is a good resource on Rick Simpson, RSO and other alternative treatments for early and late stage cancer.

RSHO(™) products are made from hemp oil with high concentrations of CBD. These products are no different from the excellent, high quality products produced by The Hemp Depot (www.TheHempDepot.org) and Charlotte's Web Hemp (www.CWhemp.com.) The similarity between names 'RSO' and 'RSHO' can cause some confusion.

Dosing

There is not enough evidence at this time to recommend using CBD in the treatment of cancer. The three mechanisms discussed above should have a positive impact on cancer, but the amount of data on use in humans is very limited at this time.

What clinical evidence is available about the use of cannabis for the treatment of cancer has been mostly done using RSO(™). This book is about CBD, and any information about RSO(™) can be obtained from the resources recommended above.

CBD can have a positive therapeutic effect on cancer-related pain, anxiety, depression and mood. Please refer to the specific chapters for these topics.

Pertinent website:

https://www.cancer.gov/about-cancer/treatment/cam/hp/cannabis-pdq

CHAPTER 22

AUTISM SPECTRUM DISORDER

Introduction:

Autism Spectrum Disorder (ASD), commonly known as autism, is a serious developmental disorder that impairs the ability to communicate and interact. The disorder varies greatly in severity and characteristics, creating a "spectrum" of skills, symptoms, and levels of disability. ASD is considered a somewhat common disorder, with over 200,000 cases a year. While females are affected by ASD, it is more common in males and is usually diagnosed during young childhood years. Seizure disorder occurs in about one third of the cases. It is felt that abnormalities can cause changes in brain activity disrupting the nerve cells in certain centers in the brain.

Until recently there was another condition called Asperger's syndrome, which was separate from Autism Disorder. However, in the latest edition of the Diagnostic and Statistical Manual of Mental Disorders (DSM-5), there are no longer subcategories, but instead just Autism Spectrum Disorder, which includes a range of characteristics and severity within one category.

Diagnosing ASD can occur reliably by the age of two. A doctor will look a child's behavior and development, as well as discuss the child's behavior with a parent. Diagnosing ASD in adults is not as simple as with young children, and the testing for adults is still being refined. Adults who may suspect ASD can speak with a psychologist or psychiatrist with ASD expertise about signs and symptoms.

While scientists and doctors don't know the exact cause of ASD, some risk factors have been identified.

According to NIMH risk factors include:

Gender—boys are more likely to be diagnosed with ASD than girls

Having a sibling with ASD

Having older parents (a mother who was 35 or older, and/or a father who was 40 or older when the baby was born)

Genetics—about 20% of children with ASD also have certain genetic conditions. Those conditions include Down syndrome, fragile X syndrome, and tuberous sclerosis among others.

In recent years, the number of children identified with ASD has increased. Experts disagree about whether this shows a true increase in ASD since the guidelines for diagnosis have changed in recent years as well. Also, many more parents and doctors now know about the disorder, so parents are more likely to have their children screened, and more doctors are able to properly diagnose ASD, even in adulthood.

There is currently no cure for ASD, but a number of therapies and treatments exist. Early treatment for ASD is crucial as it can help an individual learn new skills, make the most of their strengths, and reduce certain difficulties. In some early interventions, therapists will use highly structured and intensive training sessions to aid children in developing positive social and language skills, while discouraging negative behaviors. It has also been shown to be helpful if the family of the child with ASD participates in therapy, to help them cope with the challenges of living with someone with ASD.

Medication is another treatment options for ASD, but it does not cure or even treat the main symptoms. It can help with seizures and symptoms like obsessive compulsive disorder (OCD), depression, anxiety or severe behavioral problems. But as with many medications, sometimes the side effects of the medication are worse than the symptoms themselves.

Behavioral Symptoms

Inappropriate social interaction
Compulsive behavior
Persistent repetition of words
Impulsivity
Poor eye contact
Self-harm
Repetitive movements

Cognitive Symptoms

Problems paying attention
Intense interest in limited number of things

Developmental Symptoms

Speech delay in children
Learning disability

Psychological Symptoms

Depression
Anxiety
Unaware of others' emotions

Other Symptoms

Tics
Sensitivity to lights
Sound
Touch
Smells
Change in voice

Early indicators of ASD may include:

No babbling or pointing by age 1
No response to name
Poor eye contact
No single words by age 16 months
No two-word phrases by age 2
Excessive lining up of toys or objects
No smiling or social responsiveness

Later indicators of ASD may include:

Impaired ability to make friends or initiate/sustain
conversations with others
Repetitive or unusual use of language
Inflexible adherence to specific rituals or routines
Repetitive or unusual use of language
Absence/impairment of social or imaginative play

CBD and ASD

Considering that the symptoms and severity of ASD varies, treatment options also vary. Cannabis, particularly CBD or a combination of THC and CBD with high CBD and low THC, have been found to be effective treatments. These high CBD/low THC medications are also effective for the treatment of childhood epilepsy. CBD is also known for having both analgesic (pain reducing) and anxiolytic (anti-anxiety) effects, effectively treating many of the symptoms of ASD

In a study done by the University of California, the researchers found that "CBD regulates emotion and focus, acting as a neuroprotective against further nerve cell damage. In the autistic patient, mood can be regulated with oral doses of cannabis... CBD has reduced anxiety, rage and hostility in patients by inducing a relaxed, steady and calm demeanor. When including the positive effect of cannabis on seizures, the potential use of CBD for treatment of ASD because very real."

Dr. Adi Aran, an Israeli doctor, is currently conducting a first of its kind clinical trial involving CBD for treating autism in children and young adults. Aran was experiencing parent's asking for cannabis for their children with ASD and feeling uncomfortable prescribing something he hadn't researched, Aran conducted an observational study on 70 of his autistic patients.

The results demonstrated that CBD provided significant improvements in many of the children. Some children no longer threw tantrums or hurt themselves, while others were more communicative. It is the positive results of this observational study that has led to him conducting his two-year clinical trial.

Dosing

For those ASD patients with epilepsy, the dosing guidelines found in the seizure and epilepsy chapter should be followed.

In general CBD has been shown to be helpful for long term control of the number and severity of the seizures. Because of this use a whole plant extract that is swished inside of the front of the mouth. The starting dose is for children is ½ milligram per pound/weight, divided into three, equal, daily doses (morning, afternoon, and bedtime.) So a child weighing 100lbs would take approximately 17mg, three times a day, for a total of 50mg.) This dose can be doubled after four days to see if there is further improvement. Continue to increase by ½ milligram per pound, every four days.

So the second dose for a 100lb child would be 1mg per pound or 100mg, divided into three doses of 33mg each. Keep increasing until improvement plateaus. The maximum recommended dose is 5mg per pound a day.

THC, sometime present in "High-CBD" products. can actually aggravate epilepsy, so make certain that the products you choose are certified laboratory tested, and have low amounts of THC (less than 0.3%).

For treatment of patients with ASD without epilepsy, the most important symptoms are those of decreased social interaction, poor mood, anxiety and tantrums. CBD is safely started at ½ milligram per pound/weight, divided into three, equal, daily doses (morning, afternoon, and bedtime.) So a child weighing 100lbs would take approximately 17mg, three times a day, for a total of 50mg.) This dose can be doubled after four days to see if there is further improvement. Continue to increase by ½ milligram per pound, every four days.

So the second dose for a 100lb child would be 1mg per pound or 100mg, divided into three doses of 33mg each. Keep increasing until improvement plateaus. The maximum recommended dose is 5mg per pound a day.

Involving Medical Professionals

Childhood or adult-onset epilepsy is a significant and potentially life-threatening condition. Although it has not been reported, it is possible that the large doses of CBD required to control seizures may change the liver enzymes metabolism of prescription drugs used to treat epilepsy.

Because of the complexity and severity of seizure disorder, and possibility medication interaction with CBD or medical marijuana, patients and guardians of patients with epilepsy should always work closely with their neurologist to determine if adding CBD or medical marijuana is appropriate. The neurologists, usually have little or no training on the subject and often won't actually recommend the CBD. However, then may give their permission to add CBD to the patient's treatment.

Pertinent Website:

https://www.leafly.com/news/health/how-does-cannabis-consumption-affect-autism

CHAPTER 23

ACNE, PSORIASIS AND OTHER SKIN CONDITIONS

Personal Story

A lovely gentleman came in to see me with very red, scaly, large patches of psoriasis on his knees and elbows. He was distraught because he loved to wear shorts and a t-shirt in the warm California climate. However, he felt ugly with the large red plaques on the front of his knees and back of his elbows. He had tried several medicated creams, without much effect. He did not want to have the severe side-effects that can occur with the potent and expensive biologic medications that are advertised on TV. After a detailed history and exam, I found that he was an excellent candidate to use topical medical cannabis. Psoriasis is an inherited condition, caused by excess build up of skin cells, and causes ugly raised red patches, that are often itchy and painful. I started him of twice daily preparation of CBD and THC cannabis cream. Because the inflamed surface of his skin would more easily absorb medication into the bloodstream than healthy skin I warned him not to apply to much to the skin. He returned six weeks later wearing a t-shirt, shorts and a big smile on his face.

Introduction

The skin is the largest organ of the body. It is made of several layers each with different type cells. It also has glands that produce sweat, and hair follicles connected with glands that produce oily sebum. At the base of the layers of the skin are the cells that produce protective pigment, called melanocytes. These are when melanoma cancer starts.

Skin Condition Symptoms

Rash

Peeling skin

Ulcers

Raised bumps

Discolored patches of skin

Dry or cracked skin

Open Sores

Rough or scaly skin

The skin has many functions. It provides protection against ultraviolet light and a physical barrier that prevents chemicals and microbes from entering the body. It has several other functions related to the production of moisturizing sebum, and regulation of the body's temperature through sweat release and hair.

Under the skin layer is the subcutaneous tissue, that is very fibrotic in nature, and several conditions can result in excess fibrosis tissue formation.

Acne is a very common skin condition, especially in teenagers and in some adults with acne rosacea with over 3 million cases a year in the US. It occurs when hair follicles plug with dead skin cells and oils and can occur anywhere on the body. According to the American Academy of Dermatology acne is the most common skin condition in the United States.

Psoriasis is another very common skin conditions that also affects over 3 million Americans a year. Is is characterized by skin cells that build up and form itchy, dry patches and scales. Psoriasis, unlike acne, is an inherited autoimmune disease. It is treatable, but unfortunately not curable. The areas most commonly affected by psoriasis are the knees, scalp, and outside of elbows, but it can occur anywhere on the body. There are various severities of psoriasis.

Psoriasis is due to excess proliferation of the top layer of cells, known as keratocytes. The keratocytes have both CB1 and CB2 receptors. Cannabis-infused topical medications will decrease how fast these cells are reproducing or proliferating, and also increase the rate of programmed cell suicide, called apoptosis. The CBD, since it impacts the THCV1 receptor, will decrease the perception of itch, heat and pain that often accompanies thick psoriatic plaques.

Eczema, and atopic or irritant dermatitis are due to inflammation in the skin layers, due to allergens or chemical irritants. In addition to red, irritated skin, there is often itch, a sensation or heat or pain. These conditions respond nicely to a CBD. It activates CB1, CB2 and TRPV1. This results in decreased inflammation and swelling, and decreased perception of itch, heat and pain.

Sunburn is really just a variation of dermatitis. It is inflammation and swelling in the skin due to the effects of too much sun exposure. It responds nicely to a CBD.

Skin cells typically have both CB1 and CB2 receptors, and cannabis can be used as a preventive to decrease the damage from UVB light and inflammation and swelling after excess sun exposure. However, the use of 30+ sunblock, protective clothing, and decreasing sun or artificial UVB light exposure are primary means of preventing skin cancers and sunburn.

Insect bites result in localized inflammation, and burning sensation via the TRPV1 receptors. CBD often erases this effects of the bite immediately.

Fibrosis in the subcutaneous tissues can cause conditions such as scleroderma, Peyronie's disease of the shaft of the penis, and Dupuytren's contractures of the hand or feet (below). These tissues only have CB2 receptors. Stimulation of the CB2 receptor leads to decreased inflammation and fibrotic tissue formation.

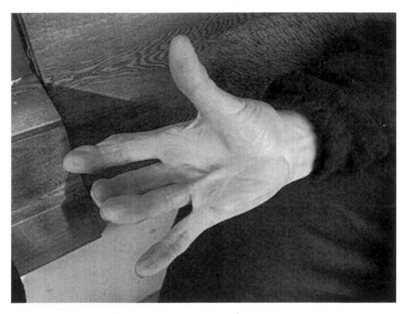

Dupuytren's of the 4th finger

Hair loss is usually due to decreased hair shaft elongation and the hair follicle going dormant. The hair follicle has CB1 receptors. Unfortunately, activation of CB1 on the hair follicle results in decreased hair shaft growth and promotes the follicle to go dormant. No cannabis-infused topical preparation is recommended.

More than any other the condition above, skin cancer (basal cell, squamous cell, or melanoma) needs to be treated under the strict supervision of a medical provider. While cannabis-infused medications may be a helpful addition to the treatment, the available evidence does not support using cannabis alone to treat skin cancer.

Considering there are so many types of skin conditions, there is also a large number of potential treatments for skin conditions. Acne, for example, can be treated with oral antibiotics, medicated soaps, topical retinoids, lotions, or contraceptives in women. Psoriasis is often treated with steroid creams, light therapy, vitamin D, or biological drugs. Other skin conditions can be managed by drugs, soaps, and paying close attention to one's lifestyle choices such as diet and exercise.

CBD Treatment

The skin cells, called keratocytes, have both CB1 and CB2 receptors. The hair follicle has only CB1 receptors. The sebaceous glands have only CB2 receptors. The subcutaneous tissue cells have only CB2 receptors. The TRPV1 receptors are found in the tiny skin nerve fibers and send the sensation of itchiness or burning to the brain.

In general patients try topical CBD preparations because the regular medications that they are using are not working, as was with the case with the gentleman in my story. Another good reason to try topical cannabis, is that the prescription medication may have severe side-effects. As you will learn, topical cannabis has only a few mild side-effects, that resolve by discontinuing the medication.

The term pruritus means itching that can occur anywhere on the body. This can be caused by bug bites, healing wounds, dry skin, or a variety of skin conditions. A study was done by S Stander, *et al.* with 22 patients experiencing itching of the skin. They were given a topical cannabinoid in the form of a cream to reduce the itching. The results of the study showed that the reduction in itching was 86.4% after the topical cream was used. The researchers concluded that topical cannabinoids, such as CBD, represent a well-tolerated and effective treatment for the reduction of itching in various conditions.

CBD has also been proven to have anti-inflammatory properties which is useful in the treatment of a certain type of skin conditions such as acne. Inflammatory acne is caused by chronic inflammation of the skin, and CBD can reduce the inflammation around pimples, which decrease the likelihood of acne spreading. However, stimulation of CB2 receptors in the follicles can increase the amount of sebum being produced, which would aggravate the acne. CBD has also been shown to have antioxidant effects, which can protect the skin from free radicals such as smoke, oils, and UV rays. Protecting the skin from these radicals can help prevent and treat various skin conditions.

Dosing

CBD has long acting effects, so initially try using the topical preparation once a day in a nice thick layer. Gently rub the medication into the skin to improve penetration into the tissues. Depending on what condition you are treating, give the once a day application a chance to work, 5-7 days before considering going to twice a day. If after two weeks of regular application you are not getting satisfactory results, consider buying a different product with a higher strength of CBD or different vehicle in the preparation. Usually, the less expensive and more popular brands will have less CBD in them, than other more expensive products.

Don't stop taking any topical medications prescribed by your doctor without consulting in advance.

There are several conditions where subcutaneous, or under the skin, fibrotic nodules result in a painful or impairing condition, or disfigurement. Dupuytren's contracture of the hand (shown in the photo above) and Peyronie's disease, which is a fibrotic contracture of the base of the penis, both respond very nicely to CBD topical. Scleroderma, is an autoimmune disease that results in a serious condition due to increased fibroblast cell activity in several organs. This also responds to long-term use of CBD. Fibroblast cells, which many CB2 receptors on them, form these scar-like tissue under the skin. Activation of the CB2 receptors with CBD results in decreased tissue fibrosis in the skin and organs, such as the liver.

Dosing Fibrotic Nodules:

For treatment of one to a few subcutaneous nodules, local application of CBD twice daily for 2-3 weeks usually results in marked reduction in nodule size, thickness and symptoms. To improve the penetration of the CBD into nodule, it is recommended that a thick portion of high-potency CBD gel or cream is used. A latex or similar glove is placed over the hand or penis. The glove seals the medicine in, and causes much more absorption deeper into the subcutaneous tissues.

Dosing for Scleroderma or Liver Fibrosis:

The goal for CBD treatment for these chronic conditions is to maintain an increased level of CB2 activation on fibroblast cells throughout the skin and organs of the body. So the treatment is 20mg three times daily, ongoing. The dose can be increased after 60 days to 30mg three times daily, if there is no effect from 20mg dose. Keep increasing the dose by 10mg, every 60 days up to maximum of 400mg.

<u>Other ingredients</u>

For the skin conditions in this chapter purchase a CBD topical that doesn't have added ingedients for muscles or joints. Many other ingredients can be added to topical medications, these include, cayenne, camphor, capsaicin, clove, wintergreen, and menthol. Most of these are essential oils that have been used for hundreds of years for topical application for sore muscles, and stiff joints. They all work by decreasing the perception of pain and inflammation. These ingredients are added when the topical preparation is being used for a local joint or muscle pain or swelling, and not for the skin conditions described in this chapter.

Treatment doesn't always work

Medicine is an art, more than it is a science. Sometimes the recommended treatment doesn't work. It may not work because the dose wasn't correct, or it may not work because the underlying condition causing the symptoms is more severe than originally thought.

Involving Medical Professionals

Skin can be a serious, and sometimes represent a more serious underlying condition in the body. Many skin conditions need to be managed by a physician. Always involve your treating physician with decisions to add CBD or medical cannabis to the treatment of serious or chronic skin conditions

<u>Pertinent Website:</u>

http://www.medicalmarijuanainc.com/cbd-hemp-oil-works-skin-care/

CHAPTER 24

PREVENTIVE DOSES OF CBD AND SAFETY

Preventive Doses of CBD

The available evidence discussed throughout this book shows that CBD raises the cannabinoid tone in the brain and body. The main net effect of using CBD on a long term basis as a preventive medicine would be decreased inflammation in many chronic degenerative disease that affect us as we age. Table I lists those diseases that have been scientifically associated with chronic inflammation.

Table I
Alzheimers and other dementias
Cardiovascular diseases such as heart attack and stroke
Inflammatory-related cancers, such as bowel, prostate, breast and lung
Autoimmune diseases, such as inflammatory arthritis, celiac disease and psoriasis

In addition, long term improved endocannabinoid tone is associated with an improved mood, reduced anxiety and perceived stress.

Finally, current societal influences on the ECS results in endocannabinoid deficiency syndromes that include: Irritable bowel syndrome, fibromyalgia, and migraine headache. This deficiency of natural ANA, would be improved by the daily use of CBD.

Safety

This book has also discussed the many studies and clinical observations that confirm the safety of CBD, even in young infants. CBD extracts really could be sold next to olive oil in a grocery store. Therefore, daily use of low doses of CBD for preventive purposes is considered safe.

Based on the above facts, I purpose a daily dose of 10-20mg a day of CBD extract, under the tongue or via vaporizer (4-8 vape inhalations a day.)

This type of preventive dosing is analogous to the U.S. Preventive Services Task Force recommendation of taking 81mg aspirin dose daily for prevention of cardiovascular disease and colorectal cancer.

Pertitent Website:

https://www.uspreventiveservicestaskforce.org/Page/Docum ent/RecommendationStatementFinal/aspirin-to-prevent-cardiovascular-disease-and-cancer

More information -

Go to www.TheHempDepot.org and use the COUPON CODE – EVD6AAT0QJ64 for 10% off purchases of whole plant, high quality CBD products.

To learn more about the author, his other books, and up-to-date research on CBD and medical cannabis go to www.Cannabis-MD.com and www.GregoryLSmithMD.com

Abbreviations

11-OH-THC- 11-Hydroxy-THC is the main active metabolite of tetrahydrocannabinol (THC) which is formed in the body after cannabis is consumed. It is more euphoric and potent than THC.

2-AG- 2-Arachidonoylglycerol is an endocannabinoid, an endogenous agonist of the CB1 receptor.

ANA- Anandamide is a fatty- acid neurotransmitter

ASD- Autism Spectrum Disorder, describes a range of conditions classified as neurodevelopment disorders

CBD- Cannabidiol is one of at least 144 active cannabinoids identified in cannabis. It is a major phytocannabinoid, accounting for up to 40% of the plant's extract in some strains.

CBG- Cannabigerol is a non-intoxicating cannabinoid found in the cannabis genus of plants.

CB1- The cannabinoid receptor type 1 is a G protein-coupled cannabinoid receptor located primarily in the central and peripheral nervous system.

CB2- The cannabinoid receptor type 2 is a G protein-coupled receptor located primarily on immune system cells. It is closely related to the cannabinoid receptor type 1.

CSA- The Controlled Substances Act is the statute establishing federal U.S. drug policy under which the manufacture, importation, possession, use, and distribution of certain substances is regulated. It was established in 1970.

FAAH- Fatty acid amide hydrolase is an enzyme. It was first shown to break down anandamide (ANA) in 1993.

FDA- The Food and Drug Administration is a federal agency of the United States Department of Health and Human

Services, one of the United States federal executive departments. The FDA is responsible for protecting and promoting public health.

FM- Fibromyalgia is a medical condition characterized by chronic widespread pain and a heightened pain response to touch. Other symptoms include fatigue to a degree that normal activities are affected, sleep problems, and troubles with memory.

GRAS- Generally recognized as safe is an FDA designation that a chemical or substance added to food is considered safe by experts, and so is exempted from the usual Federal Food, Drug, and Cosmetic Act food additive tolerance requirements.

IBD- Inflammatory bowel disease is a group of inflammatory conditions of the colon and small intestine. Crohn's disease and ulcerative colitis are the principal types of inflammatory bowel disease.

IBS- Irritable bowel syndrome is a group of symptoms-including abdominal pain and changes in the pattern of bowel movements without any evidence of underlying damage.

MDD- Major depressive disorder, also known simply as depression, is a mental disorder characterized by at least two weeks of low mood that is present across most situations. It is often accompanied by low self-esteem, loss of interest in normally enjoyable activities, low energy, and pain without a clear cause.

MS- Multiple sclerosis is a demyelinating, autoimmune disease in which the insulating covers of nerve cells in the brain and spinal cord are damaged. This damage disrupts the ability of parts of the nervous system to communicate, resulting in a range of signs and symptoms, including physical, mental, and sometimes psychiatric problems.

PEA- Palmitoylethanolamide is an endogenous fatty acid amide that stimulates receptors in the brain. PEA has been demonstrated to bind to receptors inside the cell nucleus, not on the cell membrane, and exerts a great variety of biological functions similar to CBD, related to chronic pain and inflammation.

PTSD- Post-traumatic stress disorder is a severe anxiety disorder that can develop after a person is exposed to a traumatic event, such as sexual assault, warfare, traffic collisions, or other threats on a person's life.

RA- Rheumatoid arthritis is a chronic, inherited, autoimmune disorder that primarily affects joints. It typically results in warm, swollen, and painful joints that can become disfigured in more severe cases.

RSHO- A brand of hemp oil, that is high in CBD. It is not to be confused with Rick Simpson Oil (RSO), a very potent THC-rich oil for late stage cancer.

RSO- Rick Simpson oil, also known as Phoenix Tears. This is a very potent, THC-rich oil, used in a 90-day regimen for late stage cancer. Requires a physician's supervision.

THC- Tetrahydrocannabinol refers to a psychotropic cannabinoid, and is the principal psychoactive constituent of cannabis.

TRPV1- The transient receptor potential cation channel subfamily V member 1, also known as the capsaicin receptor and the vanilloid receptor 1. It is a receptor that is important for temperature regulation and sensation of heat.

INDEX